FERTILITY

A comprehensive guide
to natural family planning

New edition

Dr Elizabeth Clubb
and Jane Knight SRN

Diagrams and charts by the Department of Medical Illustration,
John Radcliffe Hospital, Oxford

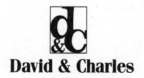

David & Charles

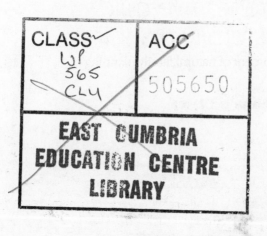

A catalogue record for this book is available from the British Library

ISBN 0-7153-0027-X

© Dr Elizabeth Clubb and Jane Knight 1987, 1992

First published 1987
Second impression 1988
Revised edition 1992

Typeset by Typesetters (Birmingham) Ltd,
Smethwick, West Midlands
and printed in Great Britain
for David & Charles Publishers plc
Brunel House   Newton Abbot   Devon

Contents

Acknowledgements

The authors would like to thank the following:

Professor John Marshall who pioneered the temperature method and established the first organisation to teach natural methods of family planning in the United Kingdom.

Professor John Bonnar for his encouragement and time spent in reading and correcting the manuscript.

Dr Cecilia Pyper and our colleagues in the Natural Family Planning Service of C.M.A.C. for their constructive criticism.

Dr Anna Flynn and her colleagues in the National Association of Natural Family Planning Teachers for their co-operation.

Dr Suzanne Parenteau-Carreau, Rita Briault and other members of SERENA, Canada who have shared their expertise in teaching fertility awareness to women after childbirth and during the difficult premenopausal years.

John and Evelyn Billings for their work in the development of the ovulation method.

Dr Peter Jones for his advice in updating the section on AIDS.

The editors of the International Review of Natural Family Planning, St John's University, Collegeville, Minnesota for their permission to use the illustrations on cervical mucus by Erik Odeblad.

The authors are very grateful for the WHO resource package to which they have made constant reference in producing this book.

Foreword

This highly readable book will be of major interest to any couple who wish to understand their fertility and to know about natural family planning methods. The book should be essential reading for any doctors or nurses who give advice on family planning. It is the most up-to-date and comprehensive handbook on natural family planning which is now available.

In the last 15 years the understanding of both fertility and infertility has greatly increased. One aspect of this has been a continuing interest in natural family planning, namely, the control of fertility based on the observation of the naturally occurring signs and symptoms of the fertile and infertile phases of the menstrual cycle and the use of this knowledge both to avoid and to achieve pregnancy. No medical scientist who is informed about the problems of present contraceptive technology throughout the World would envisage any simple and universal remedy for the problems of fertility control. Concern about the side-effects and discontinuation rates with the use of hormones and intra-uterine devices has led a number of scientists to investigate natural family planning.

Many women given the opportunity now express a strong preference for natural childbirth to allow them to give birth without drugs and medical intervention. A similar view is now being taken about birth control. Like natural childbirth, natural family planning requires a strong motivation in the couple which is fostered by education and support so that the couple have confidence in themselves and in the methods.

The current methods of natural family planning are based on the concept of fertility awareness – the woman's ability to identify on a day to day basis certain changes in her body related to the preparation for ovulation. In contrast to oral contraceptives and the intra-uterine device which usually requires the supervision of a doctor, natural family planning involves an educational and learning process rather than a medical service and aims to make the users both independent and potential educators of other users. The recent international studies of the World Health Organisation have shown that virtually all women can learn to detect the fertile and infertile times of their cycle irrespective of educational level.

Dr Elizabeth Clubb and Jane Knight provide in this book an excellent review of the current methods of natural family planning and their use in special circumstances eg following childbirth and during breast-feeding, after coming off the pill, and the pre-menopausal years. They provide in a straightforward way the factual information on human reproduction which provides the scientific basis for the cycle of fertility. Based on their firsthand experience of teaching natural family planning over many years, they deal with the problems which can arise in learning and using the methods. They discuss the latest research into natural family planning and its implications for the use of these methods.

The book also includes an up-to-date review of infertility and the application of the knowledge from natural family planning to assist in improving the chances of pregnancy. The causes of infertility and the investigations which are required in the infertile couple are dealt with in simple language. A factual account is also given of the available methods of contraception, sterilisation, abortion and sexually transmitted disease.

John Bonnar.

JOHN BONNAR, MA., MD., FRCOG.
*Professor of Obstetrics and Gynaecology
and Dean of the Faculty of Health Sciences,
Trinity College, University of Dublin.*

Introduction

Natural family planning is a method for achieving or avoiding pregnancy by observation of the natural signs and symptoms of the fertile and infertile phases of the menstrual cycle. This book describes all methods of natural family planning, teaching techniques, and the advantages and disadvantages. It can be used by medical and nursing personnel, by teachers of natural family planning and by anyone wanting reliable information.

Fertility and infertility are subjects of profound interest to scientists and to the public. The advances in research during the last 15 years have contributed to a revolution in both our knowledge and the treatment of fertility problems. The latest research proves the validity of fertility awareness techniques. This book not only covers the latest research findings but also sets them in a context that is meaningful to the lay person.

Artificial contraception, abortion, sexually transmitted diseases and related problems are best understood from a factual standpoint. This book addresses both the physiological and emotional issues giving useful background information for all those who meet these problems.

The modern awareness that a healthy life is best founded on an understanding of our own bodies is illustrated by the growing concern for balanced diet and exercise. The demand for natural childbirth, the growth of the 'Well Woman' clinics and the demand for natural methods of birth control further illustrate this. This book is designed to assist in making an informed choice about appropriate methods of family planning.

Couples who understand the natural cycle of fertility can use this knowledge to achieve pregnancy, or to space or limit their family as desired. They have the independence to control and manage their own family planning.

1 Fertility and the Development of Natural Family Planning

'The Agony and the Ecstasy' – in these words a TV documentary described the pain of infertility and the joy of giving birth. From the beginning of history the story is told how men and women sought cures for the barren wife; fertility rites and consultations with the oracle and treatments with mandragora and other herbal potions from wise women, witch doctors and the physicians of ancient times.

Today infertile couples willingly sacrifice time and money and even accept suffering undergoing treatments, to achieve pregnancy. They join long waiting lists for the privilege of being accepted on the arduous programme for in-vitro fertilisation.

Let no one say fertility is not highly prized. In many parts of the less developed world, a man's children are still his wealth. He looks to them to work for him in sickness and old age. They are his Welfare State. Family planning for him means having many children. But there is another side to this coin. As populations grow and outstrip resources, so do the social and economic pressures. In striving to live in harmony with the environment, measures to limit the size of families and of the tribe had to be taken.

From ancient times, this became apparent among peoples living in parts of the world where harsh climates prevailed and food supplies were scarce. In these lands often desperate measures were taken; infants were exposed to the elements and the old and ailing left to die, as the nomadic tribes moved on. Other populations have been controlled by laws governing the relationship between men and women, and taboos which controlled the timing and frequency of sexual intercourse.

Young couples today face social and economic problems when they assume parental responsibilities. Family planning is about having children as well as about avoiding pregnancy. It is about deciding when to start a family, the number of children and how they should be spaced, according to their circumstances.

Natural methods of family planning have been researched and developed for the purpose of finding an efficient and reliable method acceptable to peoples of different cultures and religions. The search has been to develop a method that was without health hazards and one that would help couples to conceive as well as to avoid pregnancy and therefore to be in control of their own fertility.

It is interesting to learn from World Health Organisation personnel engaged in teaching natural family planning that many peoples in Arabia, Africa, and South East Asia are aware of the rhythms of fertility and infertility occurring during the menstrual cycle. This tradition has been passed down from mother to daughter. Much of the research work has therefore resulted in rediscovery for Western civilisation of lore well known in the East.

The importance of the research work carried out during the last sixty years lies in the fact that first through the study of anatomy and physiology a scientific basis for these methods has been discovered; and secondly, that from this knowledge, accurate guidelines for identifying the fertile and infertile phases of a woman's cycle are now available.

Until the 1930s, in Western Europe, it was commonly believed that menstruation and a few days following the period were the fertile part of the cycle. Even today, many women still have misconceptions about the fertile and infertile phases of the cycle.

The Rhythm or Calendar Method
In 1929 Dr Knaus in Austria observed that ovulation occurred at a fixed time of around 14 days before the next menstrual period. In 1930 Dr Ogino in Japan, made a similar observation independently. This knowledge formed the basis of the rhythm method in which calculations were made to predict the fertile and infertile phases of the cycle. Due to its reliance on regular cycles and the long period of abstinence required, its effectiveness was poor and it was not widely accepted.

The Temperature Method
In 1928 a Dutch gynaecologist linked a rise in basal body temperature to the activity of the corpus luteum and hence to ovulation. By 1947 Ferin in Belgium suggested that the temperature rise could be used to time intercourse so as to avoid conception. In this country the practical details of the temperature method were worked out by Professor John Marshall. As use of the temperature method alone restricted intercourse to the post-ovulatory phase, he combined the temperature and calendar methods to increase the time available for intercourse.

The Mucus Method
Just as women are aware of blood flow every month during the period, so they can be helped to recognise the flow of mucus which occurs mid-

cycle. Although cervical mucus had been observed by women over the centuries, it was not until the late 19th century that Sims reported the potential of cervical mucus to block or aid sperm migration. In 1933 changes in cervical mucus were related to a rise in oestrogen levels in the urine prior to ovulation. Using mucus as an indicator of fertility and timing intercourse in relation to mucus changes was mainly the work of Drs John and Evelyn Billings in Australia. This is known as the Billings or Ovulation method of natural family planning and is widely used.

The Sympto-thermal Method

The sympto-thermal method combines observations of cervical mucus with temperature readings and other indicators of fertility. This method was variously described as the muco-thermic method (Marshall, UK) and the double-check method (Thyma, USA) It offers a high degree of effectiveness and for this reason detailed information on the sympto-thermal method and a step-by-step guide to achieve or avoid pregnancy forms the major part of this book.

The Sympto-Thermal Method

2 Reproductive Anatomy and Physiology

Some knowledge of male and female anatomy is important for each person wishing to understand natural methods of family planning. When the basic facts are clearly understood, it is easier to see how the fertile and infertile phases of the woman's cycle can be determined and why necessary rules are given.

MALE REPRODUCTIVE ORGANS

The male reproductive system is composed of two testicles (testes) from each of which runs a tube, known as the vas deferens, which opens into the urethra. The urethra is the tube which runs through the penis and conveys urine from the bladder to the outside. The seminal vesicles and ducts from the prostate gland also open into the urethra.

The testicles are contained in a special pouch of skin known as the scrotum. At puberty, they begin to function in two ways:

1. They produce the male hormone – testosterone, which is responsible for the development of male secondary sex characteristics, such as deepening of the voice, growth of the beard and pubic hair.
2. They produce male sex cells (spermatozoa, sperm). Together with the female sex cell or ovum – they are capable of producing new life.

The temperature-regulating function of the scrotum

The testes must be at a temperature slightly lower than the rest of the body, to produce sperm cells efficiently. If the temperature is too high or too low, sperm cell production is adversely affected.

The scrotum hangs outside the body, between the legs, and serves to control the temperature of the testes. If the temperature is too high, the scrotum gives off heat in two ways: by sweating; and by relaxing its muscle layer so that the surface area expands. In cold temperatures the muscle layer contracts making the surface area of the scrotum smaller and drawing the testes in closer to the warmth of the body.

Interference with the normal temperature-regulating mechanism may be a contributing factor to male infertility problems. Men working in particularly high temperatures, and men wearing excessively tight clothing, may show a low sperm count.

The production of sperm and seminal fluid

Each testis contains a long system of coiled, tightly packed tubules the linings of which produce sperm in a continuous process. The sperm then pass along to the epididymis at the upper part of the testis, where they are stored for about twelve days during which time they gain their motility and their fertilising capacity, thus reaching maturity.

At ejaculation, sperm are propelled through the vas deferens into the urethra where they join secretions from the seminal vesicles and prostate gland. These secretions assist in the preservation and nourishment of the sperm cells, and add volume to make up the seminal fluid or semen. The

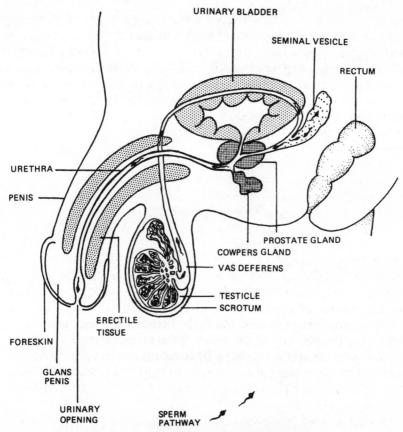

Fig 2.1 Side view of the male reproductive organs

rhythmic muscular contractions of the tubes leading from the testes to the outside, and the muscular portion of the prostate gland, help to expel the fluid with some force: ejaculation or male orgasm. Between two and five millilitres of seminal fluid containing around one hundred million sperm cells per millilitre may be thus released. Only about 100 sperm survive the long and hazardous journey to reach the ovum (female sex cell) and only one sperm will finally penetrate the ovum to achieve fertilisation and pregnancy.

The male urethra forms a common pathway for seminal fluid and urine. There is, however, a complex valve system that ensures the functions of urination and sexual activity leading to ejaculation cannot take place simultaneously.

The spermatozoon

The spermatozoon or male sex cell is microscopic in size. It comprises a head, middle section or neck and a tail. The head contains a nucleus with twenty-three rod-shaped chromosomes. These chromosomes carry the father's genes – his genetic contribution to his child. The middle section contains the energy supply to nourish the sperm and assist in movement. The slender whip-like tail enables the sperm cell to move forward by lashing energetically from side to side.

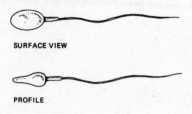

SURFACE VIEW

PROFILE

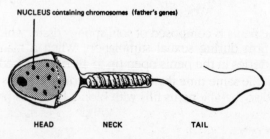

NUCLEUS containing chromosomes (father's genes)

HEAD   NECK   TAIL

Fig 2.2 Spermatozoa. The head of the sperm is ovoid-shaped but flattened, so that when seen in profile it appears pear-shaped

Mature sperm reach their full motile capacity when they are mixed with fluids from the other sex glands to form the seminal fluid or semen. This is a thick, viscous, whitish and slightly alkaline fluid with a distinct odour and acts as the medium for transporting sperm to the female genital tract.

It must be remembered that a man is always fertile. From the age of puberty (at which time sperm become mature) he may continue to produce viable sperm into the ninth decade of life.

Pre-ejaculatory fluid
The Cowpers glands secrete a lubricating fluid to prepare the urethra for sperm transport. A few drops of this fluid, containing sperm, leak out during sexual excitement and before ejaculation. It must be emphasised that even contact between male and female external genitalia, without full intercourse, could result in pregnancy in the presence of fertile mucus. The sperm may be attracted into the vagina by the mucus. For this reason coitus interruptus (withdrawal) is not a reliable means of preventing pregnancy. Even if the man withdraws in good time before he ejaculates, the pre-ejaculatory fluid containing sperm could cause a pregnancy, if there is fertile mucus present at the vaginal entrance.

Sperm survival
Sperm may survive in the female reproductive tract for up to 72 hours in the presence of fertile mucus. Longer survival times have been recorded of five or more days, but these are exceptional cases. Sperm may live in the crypts of the cervix, nourished and protected by mucus, thus retaining their capacity to fertilise the ovum.

In the absence of fertile mucus and when the cervix is forming an impenetrable barrier to sperm, that is at times of infertility, sperm remain in the vagina and are destroyed within hours by the acidity of the vaginal secretions.

The penis
The shaft of the penis is composed of soft, spongy tissue which is capable of becoming firm during sexual stimulation. When a man is sexually aroused, the arteries in the penis open up to allow increased blood-flow to the penis. At the same time the blood-flow from the penis through the veins is slowed so that the penis fills with blood, becomes firm and erect and sexual intercourse can take place. The erect penis is inserted into the vagina where ejaculation takes place.

The skin around the penis has a great number of sensitive nerve endings. These are concentrated on the underside of the shaft of the penis, and over the whole surface of the glans. When these nerve endings are stimulated, there is a build-up of sexual tension and erection of the penis. This tension is normally released at orgasm, following which the penis returns to its flaccid state. Relaxation may also occur without orgasm.

The glans penis is covered by a separate hood of skin known as the foreskin or prepuce. The foreskin retracts during erection exposing the glans. It is the foreskin which is removed at circumcision. This operation is most commonly performed for cultural or religious reasons, although there are medical reasons for circumcision.

The whole mechanism of erection and ejaculation is a reflex activity. It works most successfully in a state of relaxation. The reflex control can be affected by emotional or mental influences, drugs or alcohol. Physical or emotional stress may therefore result in a man's inability to gain or sustain an erection, and his sexual performance may be affected as a result.

FEMALE EXTERNAL GENITALIA (VULVA)

Although the major reproductive organs in the female are internal, in contrast to the external male organs, the female's external genitals are functionally important and are the counterparts of many of the male organs.

The mons pubis (pubic mound) is a soft, fatty pad lying over and pro-tecting the pubic bone. It is covered by the typically triangular shaped female pubic hair.

The mons continues backwards to form the labia majora (outer lips) of the vulva. These are soft hair-covered folds extending backwards to just in front of the anal area. They develop from the same embryological tissue as the male scrotum.

Inside the outer lips are the labia minora (inner lips) of the vulva. These are thinner and not hair-covered. They are the female counterpart of tissue that forms the shaft of the male penis. The inner lips contain numerous sensitive nerve endings. During sexual stimulation the labia become engorged with blood as does the shaft of the penis.

The labia minora unite at the front around the clitoris. The clitoris is a small knob of very sensitive erectile tissue (the female counterpart of the male glans penis). It is covered by a prepuce or hood which corresponds to the male foreskin. During sexual stimulation, by foreplay and intercourse, the clitoris enlarges by the same mechanism as does the penis, by increased blood-flow through the arteries and decreased drainage of blood from the veins. Such stimulation is important in helping a woman to achieve orgasm.

Between the clitoris and the vaginal opening lies the opening of the urethra – the urinary opening leading from the bladder.

The hymen is a thin layer of soft skin which surrounds the vaginal opening. Its size and thickness vary greatly. Many girls and young women find the hymen becomes stretched and may be relatively non-existent by the time the first act of intercourse takes place. Physical activities such as gymnastics, horse riding and the use of tampons stretch the hymen. The physical state of the hymen is not always an indicator of a girl's virginity or previous sexual experience. In a small number of women, the hymen is very thick and may cause pain on penetration in the early stages of intercourse. Very rarely, the hymen may be completely closed and may need to be opened surgically to allow menstrual blood to flow at puberty.

The area of tissue between the external genitals and the anus is known

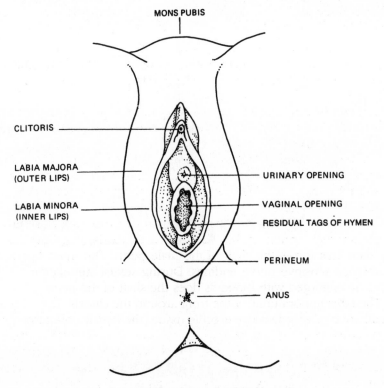

MONS PUBIS

CLITORIS

LABIA MAJORA
(OUTER LIPS)

LABIA MINORA
(INNER LIPS)

URINARY OPENING

VAGINAL OPENING

RESIDUAL TAGS OF HYMEN

PERINEUM

ANUS

Fig 2.3 Female external genitalia

as the perineum. This tissue may be damaged during childbirth. The surgical procedure of cutting the perineal tissue to enlarge the birth canal is known as episiotomy.

The external female genitalia can vary quite considerably from one woman to another. The labia minora may be quite large and often of uneven size. Women should be reassured that there is a very wide range of normality.

FEMALE REPRODUCTIVE ORGANS

The female reproductive system is composed of two ovaries from each of which runs a tube known as the fallopian tube, which opens into the cavity of the uterus. The lower end of the uterus is known as the cervix and this opens into the vagina.

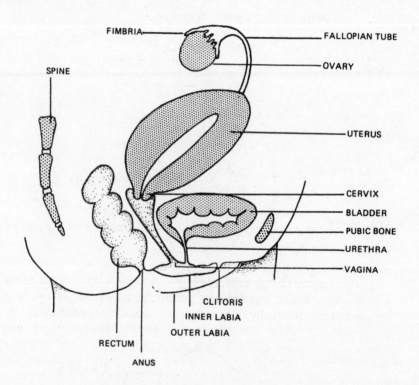

Fig 2.4 Side view of the female reproductive organs

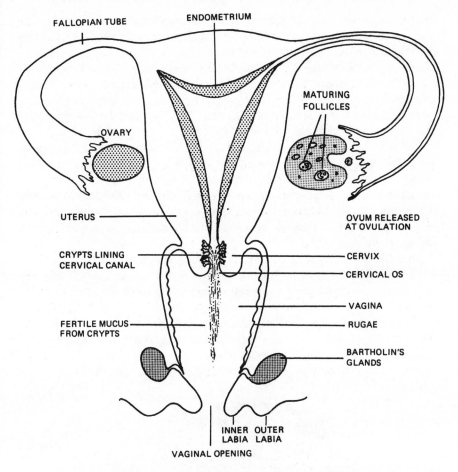

FALLOPIAN TUBE   ENDOMETRIUM

MATURING
FOLLICLES

OVARY

UTERUS

OVUM RELEASED
AT OVULATION

CRYPTS LINING
CERVICAL CANAL

CERVIX

CERVICAL OS

VAGINA

FERTILE MUCUS
FROM CRYPTS

RUGAE

BARTHOLIN'S
GLANDS

INNER OUTER
LABIA LABIA

VAGINAL OPENING

Fig 2.5 Front view of the female reproductive organs

The Ovaries

The ovaries serve two basic functions: –

1. They produce ova or egg cells, the female sex cells. In contrast to the male sperm, mature ova are not produced continuously but in a cyclical pattern. Normally only one ovum matures in each cycle.

2. The ovaries produce the female sex hormones, oestrogen and progesterone. These hormones control the menstrual cycle. They are also responsible for the development of the female secondary sex characteristics including rounding of the breasts, the growth of pubic and axillary hair.

Ovulation and the development of the corpus luteum

The ovary contains a large number of follicles. During each cycle between three and thirty follicles prepare to ripen. Each follicle forms a small fluid-filled cavity containing the ovum. Usually only one follicle will reach full maturity, which then ruptures and the ovum is released – the process of ovulation.

The ovum is the size of a pinhead. The nucleus has twenty-three chromosomes which carry the mother's genes – her genetic contribution to her child. The ovum has a lifespan of 12 to 24 hours. Thus the time after ovulation during which the ovum can be fertilised is quite short.

During the time the follicles are ripening, they produce increasing amounts of oestrogens, which are released into the blood and circulate through the body where they have an effect on various organs, including the cervix which produces cervical mucus, and the endometrium or lining of the uterus.

After ovulation, a group of cells in the ruptured follicle form the corpus luteum (yellow body) which is the flower-like structure in the ovary that produces a second hormone, progesterone. Progesterone is responsible for the rise in temperature associated with ovulation. The corpus luteum has a lifespan of 12 to 16 days, thus progesterone is effective only for a fixed length of time. Another function of progesterone is to suppress the ripening of further follicles so that if a second ovulation is to occur, it will be within 24 hours of the first. (This happens in the case of non-identical twins.)

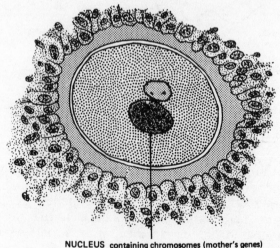

NUCLEUS containing chromosomes (mother's genes)

Fig 2.6 The ovum

The fallopian tubes and the process of fertilisation
The basic functions of the fallopian tubes are:

1. To allow the passage of mobile sperm cells.
2. To pick up the ripened ovum. The end of the fallopian tube lying adjacent to the ovary has a number of finger-like projections or fimbriae. These fimbriae create a sweeping motion which helps to pick up the ovum when it is shed from the ovary.
3. To transport the ovum towards the cavity of the uterus. The muscular action of the tube creates peristaltic waves which transport the ovum. The microscopic hairs (cilia) lining the tubes are vital to the movement of the sperm and ovum.

Fertilisation occurs when a sperm, which has travelled up through the uterus, fuses with an ovum in the outer third of the fallopian tube. The sperm must dissolve the outer coat of the ovum by a chemical reaction, to allow penetration. Immediately one sperm has done this, a chemical barrier is formed to prevent entry of any further sperm.

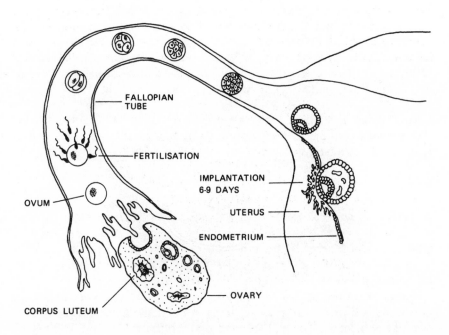

Fig 2.7 Fertilisation to implantation

The fertilised ovum or zygote receives twenty-three chromosomes from each parent, thus giving it a complement of twenty-three pairs of chromosomes – its own individual genetic structure. At this stage all the inherited characteristics are determined, for example gender, height, colour of hair and eyes.

The sex of the child is determined at the moment of conception, depending on the type of sex chromosome supplied by the sperm cell. The ovum contains twenty-two chromosomes plus one X sex chromosome. The sperm cell contains twenty-two chromosomes plus either an X or Y sex chromosome.

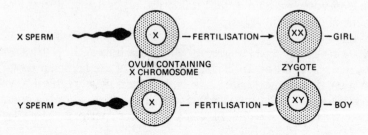

Fig 2.8 The sex of the child determined by the father

If non-identical twins are conceived as a result of two ova being fertilised separately, they may be of like sex or different sex. If identical twins are conceived, the division occurs after the ovum has been fertilised, when the genetic complement is complete. The twins will be of like sex.

The rapidly developing zygote travels along the tube and after about six days begins to embed in the nourishing lining of the uterus. This process, known as implantation, is complete about nine days after ovulation.

If the ovum is not fertilised it degenerates within 24 hours.

The uterus

The uterus is a pear-shaped organ with a thick muscular wall. It is capable of expanding greatly during pregnancy to accommodate the growing baby. During childbirth the muscular portion must generate enough force to push the infant out through the birth canal. It must then return to its normal shape and size, to prepare for another pregnancy.

The cavity of the uterus has a lining known as the endometrium. This nourishes and protects the newly fertilised egg and assists in the formation of the placenta that will serve to nourish the infant until birth.

The endometrium, because of its vital function in sustaining pregnancy, must be in good condition and to ensure this, it is completely changed each cycle. The timing of the cyclical build-up and destruction of the endometrium coincides with the release of an ovum. When an egg is ready to be fertilised, the endometrium will be ready to receive it. The maximal development of the endometrium coincides with the time when a fertilised egg would be expected to implant in the uterine cavity – about six days after ovulation.

Changes in the endometrium during the menstrual cycle

Menstruation

During menstruation, the thick soft endometrium which is rich in blood capillaries breaks down and is shed. The menstrual period lasts for three to seven days, the first days of bleeding being heavier since most of the tissue is shed at this time.

Biologically, menstruation occurs at the end of a cycle in which the ovum has not been fertilised. It is precipitated by a fall in the hormones oestrogen and progesterone. However, because the first day of menstruation is an easily recognisable landmark, for practical purposes it is taken as day one of the menstrual cycle.

The length of the menstrual cycle is obtained by counting the number of days from the first day of menstruation up to, but not including, the first day of the next menstruation. Cycle lengths vary from one woman to another, and in the same woman from one cycle to another – the common pattern being around twenty-eight days.

In anovulatory cycles, when ovulation has not occurred, the menstrual period is technically a withdrawal bleed resulting from a fall in oestrogen only, rather than a true menstrual period.

Proliferation

Following menstruation, the endometrium renews itself under oestrogen stimulation by increasing the number and size of its cells – thus becoming thicker. This phase continues until ovulation, so may be of variable length.

Secretion

Following ovulation, progesterone is produced by the corpus luteum. The endometrium has numerous mucus and sugar secreting glands which start to function under progesterone stimulation. This has a softening effect. Oestrogens continue to cause further thickening of the endometrium at this time.

If fertilisation does not occur, the corpus luteum degenerates and its hormones cease to maintain the thickened softened endometrium. The corpus luteum has an average lifespan of 12 to 16 days, after which time it is no longer active – for this reason the secretory (post-ovulatory) phase of the cycle is a fixed length of around 14 days. At the end of this phase, menstruation recurs.

If conception does occur and the fertilised ovum successfully embeds itself in the endometrium, the developing placental tissues produce the pregnancy hormone known as human chorionic gonadotrophin which maintains the life of the corpus luteum and hence the structure of the endometrium. Menstruation will not occur and the pregnancy will be sustained.

The menarche

The menarche is the first menstrual period a girl experiences, usually between 12 and 16 years.

During the first few cycles after menarche, cycle length tends to be irregular, and in quite a high proportion of cycles ovulation does not occur. Painless menstruation normally follows an anovulatory cycle. The proportion of anovulatory cycles steadily diminishes until, as reproductive maturity is reached, almost all cycles are ovulatory. Many of the early cycles where ovulation does occur have short post-ovulatory phases, and may therefore be infertile.

A young woman's cycles will normally establish themselves after several months, or a few years, into a fairly regular pattern. Cycles should only be considered irregular if they vary in length more than seven days, for example if a woman's normal cycles vary from 25 to 32 days, this is still a regular pattern.

Adolescence can provide an excellent learning experience for a young woman first introduced to the concept of fertility awareness. By observing and recording signs of her increasing maturity, a young woman can be helped to a better understanding of her cycles, and her physical and emotional changes. She may also be helped to gain respect for her body and her potential fertility.

From the time of the menarche, menstruation recurs in a cyclical pattern until a woman reaches 40–55 years of age, when the menopause marks the last menstrual period.

The cervix

The lower portion of the uterus, known as the cervix, undergoes changes during the menstrual cycle under the influence of oestrogen and progesterone. There are detectable changes in the level, position, consistency and opening of the cervix.

The cervical canal is lined with mucus membrane, forming complex crypts which secrete alkaline mucus. The lower end of the cervical canal which projects into the vagina is known as the external opening or os.

The cervix has an important role to play in pregnancy and childbirth. During pregnancy it closes off completely to protect the developing baby from the non-sterile environment of the vagina. During labour and delivery , it gradually shortens and opens to allow passage of the mature baby. After delivery, it rapidly returns to its normal size, shape and function, in preparation for the next pregnancy.

Cervical mucus
The mucus-secreting glands or crypts, lining the cervical canal, produce their fluids continuously, but the quality and quantity vary considerably throughout the cycle. The progressive changes in the characteristics of cervical mucus are under the influence of the sex hormones, oestrogen and progesterone.

During the menstrual and early pre-ovulatory phases of the cycle, when the oestrogen and progesterone levels are low, the mucus is thick and sticky. It retains its shape due to its high cellular content. It forms a plug over the cervix, preventing the entry of seminal fluid.

Approximately three to four days before ovulation the mucus changes in nature to a thin, transparent or cloudy type, under the influence of increasing oestrogens.

Around the time of ovulation, the cervical glands produce mucus which gives a characteristic slippery, lubricative sensation at the vulva. This mucus contains a gel-like substance which produces the effect of elasticity and lubrication, and may be stretched for several inches.

Fertile mucus maintains the life of sperm cells in the following ways:

1. It provides nourishment. Fertile mucus has increased amounts of water, salt, sugar and amino-acids. The odour of mucus varies throughout the cycle. Fertile mucus has a sweeter smell (and taste), compared with the slightly sour characteristics of the less fertile mucus. This reflects the changes in salt and sugar levels.
2. It changes the pH of the vagina. Fertile mucus is alkaline – this neutralises the acidic vaginal secretions and provides more favour-able conditions for sperm survival.
3. Fertile mucus aids sperm migration. The molecules of fertile mucus are arranged as long chains, or canals, through which sperm can easily pass.

Cervical mucus appears to filter out any defective sperm. There is always a proportion of immature or damaged sperm in the seminal fluid. Whereas healthy sperm make energetic forward progression through the channels of fertile mucus, damaged sperm make poor progress and actually drift sideways, where they get caught up in the thicker mucus framework, leaving the healthy ones with a chance of fertilising the ovum.

Following ovulation, as the progesterone level rises, the mucus again becomes thick and sticky, forming a plug at the cervix and preventing sperm entry.

Mucus changes can be observed by women. This forms an essential part of education in fertility awareness.

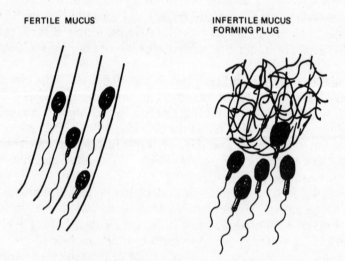

FERTILE MUCUS

INFERTILE MUCUS
FORMING PLUG

Fig 2.9 Sperm penetration in cervical mucus

The vagina

The vagina is a muscular canal leading from the cervix to the outside and is composed of an inner layer of mucus membrane and an outer muscular layer. The inner layer forms many folds or rugae, giving it a characteristic wrinkled texture. Its opening at the vulva lies between the urethra or urinary opening in front, and the anus behind.

Micro-organisms known as Doderleins or lactic-acid-producing bacillae are present in the healthy vagina. These normal vaginal inhabitants discourage the growth of bacteria which may enter the vagina from the outside. Sperm cells deteriorate rapidly in the acid environment of the vagina. They are destroyed within two to three hours, sometimes within minutes. If fertile mucus is present, its alkaline characteristics will neutralise the acid vagina, and allow sperm survival.

The muscular vaginal walls lie closely together, except during sexual excitement when there is some expansion to accommodate the erect penis. The lower end of the vagina is surrounded by a sling of voluntarily controlled muscle, which contracts to partially close the vaginal opening, and relaxes to permit entry of the penis or allow passage of the fully developed baby during childbirth. It is the strength or tone of this muscle that can be maintained (or restored after childbirth) through exercising. Good pelvic floor muscle tone can lead to improved bladder control, and support of the reproductive organs.

A healthy vagina is dependent on sufficient oestrogen. The vaginal lining changes during the menstrual cycle. If oestrogen levels are too low, there may be some dryness in the vagina, which could result in soreness and painful intercourse. This is a fairly common complaint in menopausal women.

The Bartholin's glands produce a colourless lubricative fluid in response to sexual stimulation. This is secreted around the vaginal opening to act as a lubricant in preparation for intercourse. Increased blood flow to vaginal tissues during sexual excitement also causes secretion of tissue fluid through the membranous vaginal walls. This 'arousal fluid' may be distinguished from cervical mucus because its texture is such that it cannot be stretched, unlike fertile mucus.

If a woman discovers an unusual vaginal discharge that is discoloured, has an offensive odour, or causes irritation, she should seek medical advice. Prompt treatment will prevent further problems. Her partner may also require treatment at the same time to prevent re-infection.

The sex hormone system

Hormones are chemical substances which control bodily functions. The reproductive cycle is under the control of hormones. Cycles vary in length from 23 days or less in a short cycle, to over 35 days in a long cycle. Few women have an absolutely regular menstrual cycle, and a variation of up to 7 days is perfectly normal. For convenience, we will use an average length cycle of 28 days.

First phase – pre-ovulatory, controlled by FSH and oestrogen

The pituitary gland at the base of the brain secretes FSH (follicle-stimulating hormone) which, as the name implies, stimulates the ripening of follicles in the ovary. The ripening follicles produce increasing amounts of oestrogen.

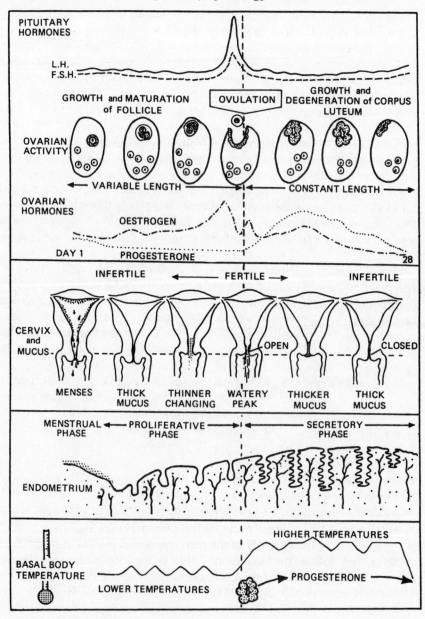

Fig 2.10 Changes during the menstrual cycle

Prior to ovulation during days 1–14 in a 28 day cycle, as the oestrogen levels rise, certain changes take place – the endometrium becomes thicker, the cervix becomes softer and the cervical mucus becomes liquid.

When the oestrogens reach a certain level in the blood, the pituitary gland is stimulated to produce a sudden surge of LH (luteinising hormone) which precipitates ovulation within 36 hours. The most mature follicle ruptures and sheds the ovum. This is ovulation.

Second phase – post-ovulatory, controlled by progesterone
Following ovulation LH causes the ruptured follicle to develop into the corpus luteum, the flower-like structure in the ovary which produces the second ovarian hormone – progesterone.

As the level of progesterone in the blood increases this causes softening of the endometrium in preparation for the implantation of a fertilised ovum. The cervical mucus becomes thick and sticky and the basal body, or resting, temperature is raised by 0.2°C or more.

The corpus luteum remains for around fourteen days, then it shrivels and dies; the level of progesterone falls; the resting temperature drops; and the endometrium degenerates, so completing the cycle. As the corpus luteum has a fixed lifespan, the interval between ovulation and the next menstruation is relatively constant within the range of 12 to 16 days. As menstrual cycles vary greatly in length, it follows that the interval between menstruation and ovulation must constitute the variable length of the cycle.

The fertility cycle
The female cycle is generally known as the menstrual cycle, menstruation being the most prominent feature of the cycle; however for purposes of fertility awareness, the cycle is often referred to as the fertility cycle, placing the emphasis on the cyclic changes of fertility.

Figure 2.11 shows an average fertility cycle of 28 days. The first day of menstruation is day 1 of the cycle. Subsequent days are numbered up to but not including the first day of the next menstrual period. A number of infertile days follow menstruation – this is the pre-ovulatory infertile phase. The fertile phase of the cycle occurs either side of ovulation. The first sign of cervical mucus heralds the onset of the fertile phase, because sperm can survive in fertile mucus awaiting ovulation. After ovulation, time must be allowed for ovum survival and the possibility of a second ovulation occurring within 24 hours. The post-ovulatory infertile phase is confirmed by a combination of temperature and mucus signs about three

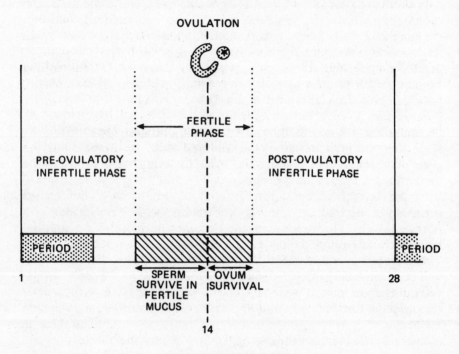

Fig 2.11 The fertility cycle

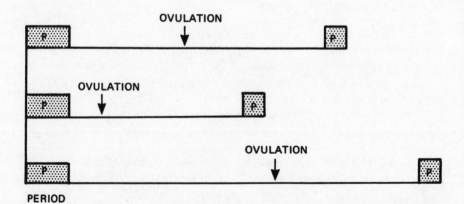

PERIOD

Fig 2.12 Normal length, short and long cycles. Note that the interval between ovulation and the next menstrual period remains fairly constant (around 14 days)

days after ovulation. This phase lasts until the onset of the next menstrual period.

Figure 2.12 shows the variation in cycle length. The interval between ovulation and the next menstrual period remains fairly constant, the normal range being 12–16 days. Cycle lengths differ because of the variable length of the pre-ovulatory phase. In a short cycle of 21 days, ovulation will occur around day 7 and there will be no pre-ovulatory infertile days. A normal length cycle (around 28 days) will have a few early infertile days and a long cycle (for example 35 days) where ovulation does not occur until around day 21, will have many early infertile days.

An understanding of fertility awareness allows a couple to determine the fertile and infertile phases of the cycle and thereby achieve or avoid pregnancy as desired. Tuition is given by doctors and nurses and also by couples who use the method and who have attended a teacher training course.

Instruction will first be given in charting the basal body temperature. This is known as the temperature method. Secondly, mucus recognition will be taught using the cervical mucus or ovulation method. Thirdly, by recording cycle lengths, a formula can be applied which is derived from the calendar method. Instruction in self-examination of the cervix is optional.

Each of these three indicators can be used as a method on their own or they may be combined to form the sympto-thermal method. First we will look at the changes in the basal body temperature, the temperature method.

3 The Temperature Method

Progesterone secreted from the corpus luteum following ovulation raises the basal body (resting) temperature by around 0.2°C and maintains it at the higher level until the time of the next menstruation. This forms the basis of recording temperature changes as an indication that ovulation has occurred. Temperature readings have no value in predicting ovulation.

RECORDING AND CHARTING THE BASAL BODY TEMPERATURE (BBT)

A special fertility thermometer is used which covers only the range from 35–39°C. This makes it easier to detect the minimal changes which occur. A woman should have two thermometers available in case of breakage. The use of a new thermometer should be recorded.

1. The mercury should be shaken down below 35°C the night before.
2. The temperature should be taken immediately on waking before getting out of bed, drinking tea or any other activity, and at about the same time each morning. If the recording time varies by more than 1 hour, this must be noted.
3. The temperature may be taken by the mouth, vaginal or rectal routes.

   a) Mouth or oral route. The bulb of the thermometer is placed under the tongue, with the lips closed and left for five minutes, in contact with the floor of the mouth.
   b) Vaginal route. The thermometer is inserted into the vagina for three minutes.
   c) Rectal route. A trace of vaseline or KY jelly is smeared on the bulb which is inserted into the rectum for three minutes, while lying on one side with the knees drawn up.

   For accuracy, whatever route has been chosen should be followed throughout the cycle. Oral temperatures can give satisfactory results if exact instructions are followed, but internal temperatures are more reliable.
4. The chart is marked with the thermometer reading by a dot in the centre of the appropriate square. If the mercury stops between two

marks the lower reading should be recorded. The dots should be joined to form a continuous graph.

5. The thermometer should be cleaned with cottonwool and cold water, (never hot water). A fertility thermometer should not be used if a fever is suspected because a high temperature may break the mercury column.
6. The first day of menstruation is Day 1 of the cycle. A new chart is started on that day. If menstruation starts during the day, that morning's temperature should be transferred to a new chart.
7. Anything unusual should be noted on the chart, such as a cold, a late night, drinking alcohol, or any stressful situation.

Digital thermometers

Many women now prefer to use battery-operated digital thermometers. Although these are more expensive, they are virtually unbreakable. They are easy to read and recording time is reduced to about one minute, whichever route is used. There is no restriction on air travel, compared with mercury thermometers which are banned on aircraft.

INTERPRETING THE TEMPERATURE READINGS

Ovulatory cycles

A cycle in which ovulation has occurred is characterised by a biphasic temperature chart. The temperature remains at the lower level until the time of ovulation, when a rise or shift occurs of about 0.2°C or more. The rise usually takes place abruptly between one day and the next. The temperature remains on the higher level until just before, or at the onset of, the next period (see fig. 3.1).

To determine the post-ovulatory infertile phase

If pregnancy is to be avoided, intercourse cannot be resumed immediately the temperature shift is recorded. The ovum can be fertilised for up to 12 hours after ovulation and allowance must be made for the possibility of a second ovulation within 24 hours of the first, a rare phenomenon which occurs in twin pregnancies.

Rule of 3 over 6

The post-ovulatory infertile phase begins after the third high temperature has been recorded. There must be three consecutive undisturbed high

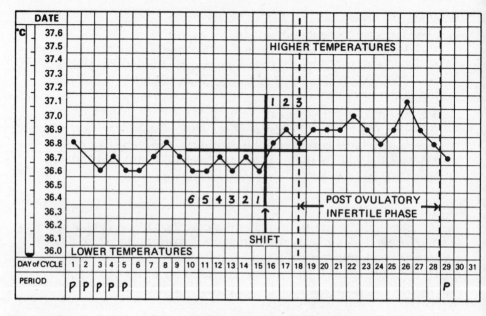

Fig 3.1 Biphasic chart showing rule of 3 over 6

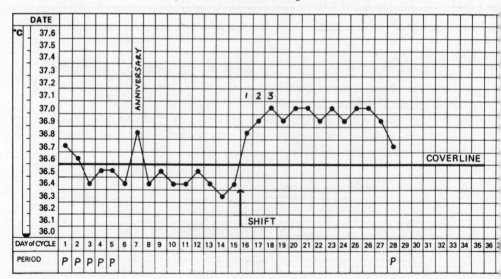

Fig 3.2 Use of a coverline

temperatures above the level of the previous six consecutive daily temperatures. The shift need only be 0.1°C but one of the three high temperatures should be at least 0.2°C above the coverline.

To identify the relevant temperatures when applying the rule of 3 over 6, a horizontal coverline is drawn on the line immediately above the highest of the low temperatures. A vertical line is then drawn forming a cross on the chart between the two days when the temperature shift from the lower to the higher phase occurred. This is illustrated in figure 3.1 with the three higher temperatures in the upper right quadrant and the previous six in the lower left quadrant. As soon as the third high temperature has been recorded, intercourse can be resumed and the rest of the cycle will be infertile.

Use of a coverline

Some organisations may use slightly different criteria for defining the temperature shift. A horizontal coverline is drawn over the low phase temperatures excluding the first four and any disturbances. The three high temperatures must all be above the coverline as illustrated in figure 3.2. The coverline technique may sometimes prove useful when interpreting a difficult chart particularly in special circumstances, but the 3 over 6 rule is very efficient and simple to apply and for this reason is the method adopted here for chart interpretation.

Variations in the temperature rise or shift

An abrupt rise is the most common with temperature showing a sharp

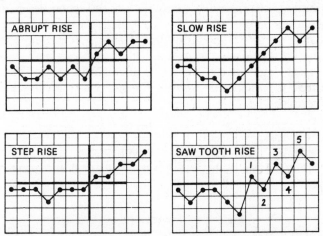

Fig 3.3 Variations in the temperature shift

rise between one day and the next, although other variations may occur less commonly.

A **slow rise** is one in which the temperature rises slowly over several days whereas a **step rise** is seen to go up in a series of steps. These are shown in figure 3.3 and may easily be interpreted using the rule of 3 over 6.

A **saw-tooth rise** goes through a series of peaks and troughs and although very rare is more difficult to interpret. By drawing a coverline, identify the beginning of the rise. The post-ovulatory infertile phase begins after the fifth temperature has been recorded as in figure 3.3.

Variations in shift day

Cycle lengths will vary considerably, but as the temperature shift occurs 12–16 days before the next period it will be apparent that it will occur earlier in shorter cycles and later in longer cycles as demonstrated in figure 3.4. The length of the pre-ovulatory infertile phase will vary accordingly but the post-ovulatory infertile phase will remain constant.

A spike

A temperature spike is defined as a single recording which is 0.2°C or more above its immediate neighbours as in figure 3.5. A spike may result from a disturbance caused by drinking alcohol, a late night, oversleeping, minor illness or stress. Sometimes there may be no obvious cause for a spike.

One temperature spike may safely be ignored when determining the six temperatures on the lower level, but where possible there should be an explanation for the temperature disturbance. If more than one spike is present, then it is advisable to wait a further few days until the position becomes clear again. If a disturbance affects one of the three higher temperatures, it is advisable to wait for a fourth high temperature to ensure infertility.

Short post-ovulatory phase

Some women will experience cycles with a shortened post-ovulatory phase, as in figure 3.6. If the post-ovulatory or luteal phase lasts less than nine days, the cycle will be infertile as there is insufficient time for implantation to take place.

Anovulatory cycles

In a small proportion of cycles, ovulation does not occur. These anovu-

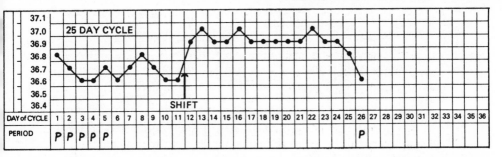

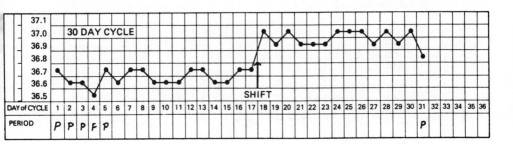

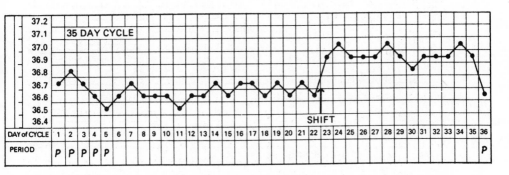

Fig 3.4 Variations in shift day

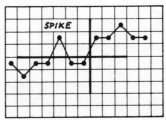

Fig 3.5 Disturbance producing a spike

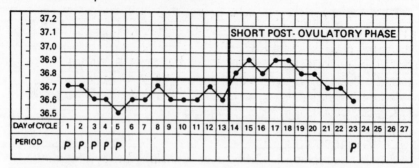

Fig 3.6 Short post-ovulatory phase

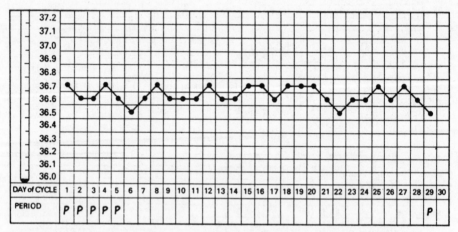

Fig 3.7 Monophasic chart indicating anovulatory cycle. Note absence of shift in temperature level

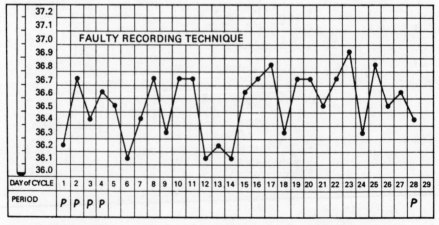

Fig 3.8 Erratic temperature readings with large swings due to faulty recording technique

latory cycles are characterised by a monophasic chart, that is the temperature readings remain on one level throughout the cycle as shown in figure 3.7. This may be contrasted with the distinct biphasic pattern demonstrated by the ovulatory cycle in figure 3.6. Anovulatory cycles are more common at the two extremes of the fertile life, adolescence and the pre-menopause. They may also occur after childbirth and after coming off the contraceptive pill.

Faulty recording technique
A very erratic temperature chart may indicate faulty recording technique as in figure 3.8. It differs from a chart affected by illness, by showing frequent subnormal readings as well as high readings. Erratic temperature readings may be seen during the learning period. It is important to ensure that temperature-taking and recording techniques are thoroughly understood. Common errors include not leaving the thermometer in place for the required length of time and not shaking the mercury down properly. If the temperature is being taken orally, it may be wise to change to the vaginal or rectal route at the beginning of the next cycle, if this is acceptable. This tends to give a more stable pattern which is easier to interpret.

4 The Cervical Mucus Method

During the menstrual cycle changes take place in the mucus produced by the glands or crypts in the cervix. These changes have been observed and their significance understood over the centuries by certain tribes in Africa and peoples in Southern Asia. Many women in western countries notice the mucus symptom, but are unaware of its significance.

REBECCA: Rebecca is an art student, living in a hostel. For some months she had been worried about a discharge that seemed to come every few weeks and lasted four or five days. When she heard a speaker on 'Fertility Awareness' at a college meeting she heaved a sigh of relief. Not only was the discharge normal, but mucus recognition would be easy.

RECOGNITION OF CERVICAL MUCUS

Mucus will be recognised by sensation and by appearance and by testing with the finger.

Sensation

Sensation is very important and the most difficult to learn. Throughout the day the presence or absence of mucus will be recognised by the sensation at the vulva, the way the beginning of a period is noticed.

Appearance

The appearance of the mucus is equally important. Soft white toilet tissue should be used to blot or wipe the vulva. There may be dampness only on the tissue resulting from the moistness associated with the vagina. This moistness soaks into the tissue and any mucus will appear raised as a blob on the tissue.

The colour should be noted. It may be transparent or opaque, creamy, yellowish or white. Mucus may be detected on underclothing, where it may have dried slightly causing some alteration in its characteristics.

Finger Testing

A finger is lightly applied to the mucus on the tissue and then pulled

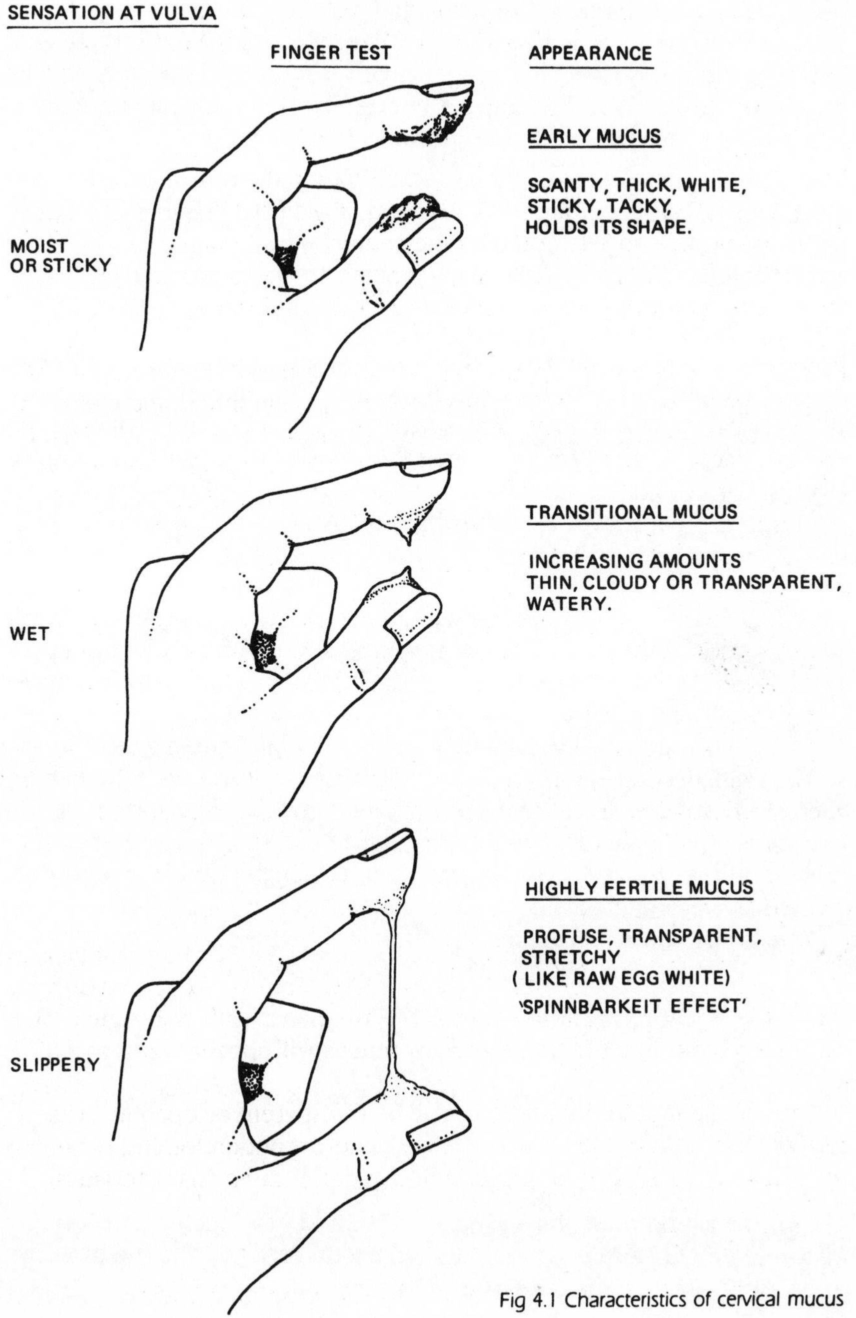

SENSATION AT VULVA

FINGER TEST

APPEARANCE

EARLY MUCUS

SCANTY, THICK, WHITE,
STICKY, TACKY,
HOLDS ITS SHAPE.

MOIST
OR STICKY

TRANSITIONAL MUCUS

INCREASING AMOUNTS
THIN, CLOUDY OR TRANSPARENT,
WATERY.

WET

HIGHLY FERTILE MUCUS

PROFUSE, TRANSPARENT,
STRETCHY
(LIKE RAW EGG WHITE)
'SPINNBARKEIT EFFECT'

SLIPPERY

Fig 4.1 Characteristics of cervical mucus

gently away to test its capacity to stretch. It may feel sticky or crumbly and break easily, or it may feel slippery like raw egg white and stretch between the thumb and first finger, from a little up to several inches before it breaks. This stretchiness is described as the Spinnbarkeit or Spinn effect, and shows that the mucus is highly fertile.

CHANGES IN CERVICAL MUCUS DURING THE FERTILITY CYCLE

Pre-ovulatory infertile dry days
Following the menstrual period there may be several dry days. These days may be absent in short cycles and numerous in long cycles. At this time the cervical mucus is thick and sticky and forms a plug blocking the cervical canal. It acts as an impenetrable barrier to sperm. A feeling of dryness or a positive sensation of nothingness at the vulva will be experienced. There will be no visible mucus.

The fertile phase
As ovulation approaches, mucus will appear in the vagina. At first it will give a sensation of moistness or stickiness at the vulva and will appear thick, white, yellow or cloudy coloured, and scanty. On finger testing the mucus will break easily.

As the oestrogen levels continue to rise with approaching ovulation, the mucus will become more profuse, and there may be up to a tenfold increase in volume. It will give a sensation of lubrication or slipperiness at the vulva. The appearance will be similar to that of raw egg white, thin, watery and transparent. On finger-testing this highly fertile mucus may stretch for several inches before it breaks.

The fertile mucus maintains the life of the sperm, nourishes it and allows it to pass through the cervix. In fertile mucus, sperm may live for up to three days, in extreme circumstances for five days or even longer.

Peak day
Peak day denotes the LAST day on which this highly fertile-type mucus is either seen or felt.

Guidelines for achieving pregnancy
Couples wishing to achieve pregnancy should have intercourse on any day when highly fertile-type mucus is present. Peak day and the two days preceding peak are the days of maximum fertility.

Post-ovulatory infertile dry days

During the post-ovulatory phase, the slippery sensation is lost and there will be a relatively abrupt return to stickiness, then later dryness again. The mucus forms a plug at the cervix acting as a barrier to sperm.

The amount and quality of mucus will vary from woman to woman and also from one cycle to the next. A woman should be alert to any changes in sensation and to even relatively small amounts of mucus.

If a woman is finding difficulty detecting mucus externally, it is often recognised more easily after a bowel movement. It may also help to use the Kegel exercise (see page 52) or a slight bearing down action to expel any mucus.

Detection of mucus in the first cycle of charting

During the first cycle of the learning period, a couple should abstain from intercourse completely until the late infertile phase has been confirmed by the instructor. This allows a woman to familiarise herself with both the change from dryness as the mucus first appears and the progressive change in her mucus pattern, without possible confusion from either seminal or arousal fluids.

Guidelines for avoiding pregnancy

Dry days following the period are infertile. Any change from the sensation of true dryness or any visible mucus warns of approaching ovulation and should be regarded as fertile.

If a woman is relying on mucus signs alone, the post-ovulatory infertile phase starts on the fourth evening past peak day. This interval allows for the fact that peak day does not coincide precisely with the day of ovulation. It allows for the life of the ovum and makes provision for a second ovulation.

THE OVULATION METHOD (MUCUS METHOD)

Doctors John and Evelyn Billings have developed earlier scientific knowledge of mucus changes into a practical method where, by observation of mucus signs alone, a woman can be aware of her natural fertility and use the knowledge to achieve or avoid pregnancy. They have their own method of charting and rules. This is commonly known as the Billings method, and is used by many people throughout the world. It is the method of choice in many of the developing countries.

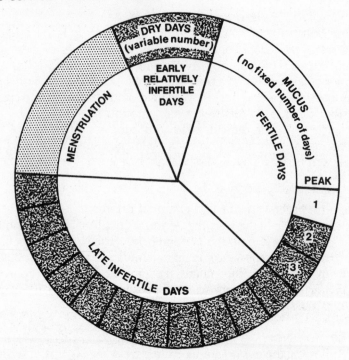

Fig 4.2 The mucus pattern of fertility and infertility (Billings)

Proponents of the Billings method would contend that inclusion of other indicators, such as temperature, causes unnecessary confusion. This has not been the experience of other NFP teachers.

Professor Thomas Hilgers in the USA has devised a scoring system to grade different types of mucus according to characteristics of sensation, colour and consistency. This is similar to the scoring system used in fertility clinics. Many women use this method effectively, relying on mucus signs alone. It requires a full programme of instruction by a qualified teacher of the method.

RECORDING MUCUS ON THE SYMPTO-THERMAL CHART

Women are taught mucus recognition as a double check with the temperature recording in the sympto-thermal method.

1. Mucus should be observed throughout the day and the chart marked each evening. This allows changes to become apparent during the day.

2. Each day of menstruation or blood loss, including spotting, is marked in red or with a P (period).

3. Each dry day when there is a dry sensation at the vulva, and no visible mucus, is marked in green or with a D.

4. Each day when there is mucus present can be marked in yellow. Days of sticky white/yellow mucus should be marked with an M and days of highly fertile-type slippery transparent stretchy mucus should be marked with an F.

5. A woman should describe the mucus in her own words.
   a) Sensation: eg moist, sticky, wet, lubricative, slippery.
   b) Observation of colour on soft, white toilet tissue: eg white, yellow, cloudy, or crystal clear. Fertile-type mucus may be blood-tinged, giving the appearance of the start of a period. This must not be misconstrued.
   c) The finger-test. Consistency may be described as crumbly, tacky, thready, or stretchy.
   In practice the characteristic mucus changes may not be well defined. There may be a combination of two types of mucus, eg cloudy, thready mucus with some transparent stretchy mucus. The mucus possessing the more fertile characteristic should be recorded.

6. Peak day is marked with a cross (X). Remember that peak day denotes the LAST day of lubricative sensation when the fertile, slippery, transparent, stretchy mucus is present. This is not necessarily the day of the most profuse mucus. The peak day will only be known in retrospect, the day following peak there will be a change to the thick, white, sticky mucus again, or to dryness.

7. The days after peak day are numbered 1, 2, 3, 4.

8. Anything unusual must be recorded on the chart, such as a late night, alcohol, stress, illness or a change in routine.

9. Any additional signs, that may indicate fertility, are recorded, for example one-sided abdominal pain, bloated abdomen, rectal pressure, or mood variations including increased libido.

10. Each act of intercourse is marked with an I. If avoiding pregnancy the significant acts of intercourse to be recorded are the last before, and the first act after the fertile phase.

11. The first fertile day should be marked with a bar (–).

Recording the mucus pattern

DAY of CYCLE	1	2	3	4	5	6	7	8	9	10	11	12	13	14	15	16	17	18	19	20	21	22	23	24	25	26	27	28	29	30
PERIOD and MUCUS	P	P	P	P	P	D	D	D																					P	

(days 6, 7, 8 marked: DRY, NOTHING / DRY, NOTHING / DRY, NOTHING)

Fig 4.3 The period and dry days – 28 day cycle
The first day of menstruation is the first day of the cycle. A variable number of dry days marked D may follow the period

DAY of CYCLE	1	2	3	4	5	6	7	8	9	10	11	12	13	14	15	16	17	18	19	20	21	22	23	24	25	26	27	28
PERIOD and MUCUS	P	P	P	P	P	M	M																			P		

(days 6, 7 marked: MOIST, WHITE, STICKY / MOIST, WHITE, STICKY)

Fig 4.4 Onset of mucus immediately after period – 25 day cycle
Wet days marked M indicate the presence of mucus and the absence of pre-ovulatory dry days. This is more common in short cycles

DAY of CYCLE	1	2	3	4	5	6	7	8	9	10	11	12	13	14	15	16	17	18	19	20	21	22	23	24	25	26	27	28	29	30
PERIOD and MUCUS	P	P	P	P	P	D	D	M	M	M																		P		

(days 8, 9, 10 marked: MOIST, WHITE, STICKY / MOIST, WHITE, STICKY / WET, CLOUDY)

Fig 4.5 Onset of mucus after dry days – 27 day cycle
Dry days marked D are followed by the onset of mucus on day 8. A woman must familiarise herself with the change in sensation from true dryness to moistness associated with the first appearance of mucus at the vulva

INTERCOURSE
↓

DAY of CYCLE	1	2	3	4	5	6	⑦	8	9	10	11
PERIOD and MUCUS	P	P	P	P	P	D	D	M	D	D	

Fig 4.6 Recording a wet day the day after intercourse in the pre-ovulatory phase. During the learning period the day after intercourse is marked as wet (M) because of the difficulty in distinguishing mucus from seminal fluid

Note: Intercourse in the early dry days is unlikely to be followed by pregnancy although intercourse in the pre-ovulatory phase always carries with it some risk.

DAY of CYCLE	1	2	3	4	5	6	7	8	9	10	11	12	13	14	15
PERIOD and MUCUS	P	P	P	P	P	D	D	M	M	M	M	F	F	✗	M
								LITTLE, WHITE	MOIST, "	STICKY, "	" CLOUDY	SLIPPERY, STRETCHY	CLEAR, "	" "	STICKY, WHITE

Fig 4.7 Mucus pattern approaching peak day. Any days of highly fertile clear stretchy mucus giving a slippery sensation are marked with an F. The last F day is peak day and is marked with a cross through the F

Fig 4.8 Peak day and the change after peak. After peak day, there is an abrupt change to sticky mucus or dryness. Four days marked 1, 2, 3, 4, must elapse before intercourse is resumed on the evening of the fourth day

12	13	14	15	16	17	⑱	19	20	21	22	23	24	25	26	27	28	29	30
F	F	✗	M 1	M 2	M 3	D 4	D	D	D	D	D	D	D	D	D	D	D	P
SLIPPERY, STRETCHY	CLEAR "	" "	STICKY, WHITE	" "	WHITE, CRUMBLY													

DAY of CYCLE	1	2	3	4	5	6	7	8	9	10	11	12	13	14	15	16	17	18	19	20	21	22	23	24	25	26	27	28	29	30
PERIOD and MUCUS	P	P	P	P	P	D	D	M	M	M	M	F	F	✗	M 1	M 2	M 3	D 4	D	D	D	D	D	D	D	D	D	D	D	P
								LITTLE, WHITE	MOIST, "	STICKY, "	" CLOUDY	CLEAR, STRETCHY	"		SLIPPERY, CLEAR	STICKY, WHITE	"	WHITE, CRUMBLY											

Fig 4.9 Mucus changes through cycle. Complete cycle showing typical pattern of menstruation, pre-ovulatory dry days, mucus days approaching peak, the count of four after peak day and post-ovulatory dry days

P–D

The sympto-thermal chart

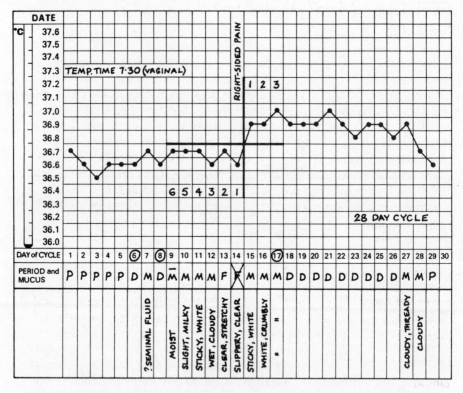

Fig 4.10 Combining the mucus and temperature recordings on the sympto-thermal chart. The chart shows a 28 day cycle with a 5 day period. The first mucus appears on day 9, this is marked with a bar to show the beginning of the fertile phase. Peak day is day 14 and the temperature shift follows between day 14 and 15.

The mucus on day 27 and 28 is related to hormonal fluctuations prior to the next period. Mucus occurring during the post-ovulatory infertile phase can be disregarded.

The couple are using fertility awareness to avoid pregnancy. They had intercourse on alternate dry days 6 and 8 and then abstained until the post-ovulatory infertile phase was confirmed by the third high temperature past peak day, on day 17. The rest of the cycle was then available for unrestricted intercourse.

CHECKLIST FOR WOMEN EXPERIENCING DIFFICULTY DISTINGUISHING CERVICAL MUCUS

Some women may have considerable difficulty determining changes in sensation, or distinguishing mucus changes; others may have a continuous discharge confusing the picture. Women in developing countries apparently have no difficulty distinguishing mucus externally. They tend to wear loose clothes, often with no underwear, and so the sensation of mucus at the vulva is experienced and is easily interpreted.

To ensure normal sensation at the vulva, and to keep the area cool, pants should be all-cotton, as they are more absorbent and cooler. Nylon tights and other synthetic underclothing should be avoided.

It is essential to maintain normal hygiene of the genital area but baby soap, or simple, non-allergic soap should be used. Perfumed or coloured soaps and even bath oils or salts may cause minor allergic reactions of the delicate skin at the vulva. Some women may be allergic to certain washing powders, or to fabric softeners. Pants should be washed in mild soap powder only. Talcum powder, vaginal deodorants and douches should never be used. These products may neutralise the acid medium and destroy the normal flora inhabiting the vagina, hence the normal self-cleansing mechanism of the vagina will be lost.

The way in which a woman deals with her menstrual bleeding may also affect her ability to distinguish mucus. It is advisable not to use internal tampons when the menstrual flow is very light, as they may cause some drying of the vagina, and the normal flora of the vagina may be removed along with the tampon. This may cause a reactive discharge from the vaginal walls.

Finally, it has been found that overwork and stress may also predispose to vaginal discharges. Good general health and dietary habits will help to maintain the normal health of the vagina. An alteration in various practices of hygiene or clothing, or attention to diet and general health and fitness, may be all that is necessary to reduce minor vaginal discharges so that cervical mucus is more easily identified.

Glass of water test

Some women find it difficult to differentiate vaginal secretions from cervical mucus. The 'glass of water test' has been devised: two fingers are used to test the secretions and are inserted into a glass of water. True mucus is insoluble and will form a blob, falling to the bottom of the glass. Vaginal secretions will disperse.

THE KEGEL EXERCISE – AS AN AID TO FERTILITY AWARENESS

This simple exercise is performed by alternately contracting and relaxing the pelvic floor muscles (around the entrance to the vagina).

To help identify these muscles, a woman can practice by using them to stop a flow of urine mid-stream. A further useful exercise is to insert one or two fingers into the vagina, then try to contract the muscles strongly, to grip the fingers, then relax.

The Kegel exercise forms the basis of antenatal exercises designed to improve pelvic tone in preparation for childbirth. It is also used as part of the postnatal exercise programme to strengthen the pelvic floor muscles which have been subject to considerable stress during pregnancy and childbirth. The exercise can be a valuable aid to fertility awareness.

The Kegel exercise will help to increase awareness of the sensation at the vulva, when performed periodically during the normal course of the day. The way in which the labia separate is most important in determining the presence or absence of cervical mucus.

The pelvic floor muscles are first contracted, then relaxed. If there is no mucus present, the labia feel dry, giving a positive sensation of 'nothingness'. If sticky mucus is present, the inner labia separate in a sticky fashion and if slippery, lubricative mucus is present, the labia slide smoothly away from one another.

If the Kegel exercise is performed effectively, then with experience, a woman will be able to identify true dryness or the presence of mucus on the day following intercourse. This experience is invaluable in the pre-ovulatory phase of the cycle, as it overrides the need for restricting intercourse to alternate evenings.

As an added bonus, a woman who has good control of the pelvic floor muscles may find increased pleasure during lovemaking. With her ability to contract these muscles strongly as desired, a woman may increase her partner's pleasure, and achieve her own orgasm more easily.

5 Factors Affecting the Menstrual Cycle

DISTURBANCES AFFECTING THE SYMPTO-THERMAL CHART

Any disturbance or change from normal routine must be noted on the sympto-thermal chart so that their effect on the cycle can be ascertained.

A disturbed night's sleep may affect the following morning's temperature reading but provided the temperature is taken after at least 3 hours rest in bed, the recording is usually accurate. A late night and alcohol may affect the temperature, giving a false high or low reading, depending on the individual.

Rising later in the morning may affect the temperature. It is generally noted that the basal body temperature rises by about 0.1°C per hour, so that taking the temperature at 9am instead of the usual 7am will increase it by 0.2°C. Likewise if the temperature is taken much earlier than usual it will be correspondingly lower. Professor Marshall recommends that for those women on shift work with varied sleep patterns, the temperature should be taken at the same time each day, irrespective of rest periods. If night work is prolonged, it may be advisable to take the temperature on waking after the longest sleep period.

Illnesses may cause a rise in temperature or pyrexia. However this rise will be much higher than the rise which occurs at the time of ovulation and so should not cause confusion in interpreting the temperature chart.

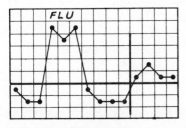

Fig 5.1 Pyrexia in the pre-ovulatory phase

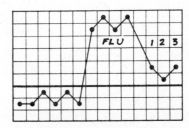

Fig 5.2 Pyrexia around the time of ovulation

If pyrexia occurs in the pre-ovulatory phase and is over before ovulation, the temperature will return to the low level and the ovulation shift will be observed later as in figure 5.1. However if the pyrexia occurs around the time of ovulation, the temperature may be seen to fall to the level of the higher phase temperatures, indicating that the ovulation shift occurred during the illness, as in figure 5.2. The woman's normal coverline can be used to help determine the position in the cycle.

Holidays and travel may delay or suppress ovulation. Air travel which involves crossing time-zones and upsets the body's natural rhythm is likely to make reliable temperature recordings impossible. It may take about a week for the body to adapt to such changes. A holiday proved to be the problem in the following case.

AMANDA AND STEPHEN: 'I really don't want to be sterilised' said Amanda. 'I am only 26 and we may want another baby in a year or two'.

Amanda suffered from allergies; barrier methods were out, the coil had caused her severe backache and very heavy periods, and she felt unwell on the pill. She and Stephen went to a class to learn about natural methods. Amanda's cycles were regular, mucus signs were recognised in the first month and her temperature charts were classical.

Then came the holiday of a lifetime on a Greek Island. Amanda accidentally left her thermometer and charts at home. 'Never mind' she told Stephen, 'We can rely on mucus signs'. Amanda discovered she was pregnant two weeks later. Relying solely on mucus signs was not so easy for her when half the day was spent in the sea. Amanda told her friends about natural methods, but her enthusiasm did not carry conviction!

A comprehensive checklist is given below of disturbances which may affect the sympto-thermal chart. This can be used as an aid to chart interpretation.

Alcohol	Holidays	Illness	Stress
Late night	Travel	Feverish cold	Drugs
Disturbed night	Time zones	Migraine	
Oversleeping	Shift work	Cystitis	
Cold in bed			

THE POSSIBLE EFFECTS OF STRESS ON THE CYCLE

Women using natural family planning should be aware of the effect stress may have on the cycle. It may affect hormonal control and ovarian

DAY of CYCLE	1	2	3	4	5	6	⑦	8	9	10	11	12	13	14	15	16	17	18	19	20	㉑	22	23	24	25	26	27	28	29	30	31
PERIOD and MUCUS	P	P	P	P	P	D	D	M	M	M	D	D	M	M	M	F	✗	M I	M 2	M 3	D 4	D	D	D	D	D	D	D	D	D	P

Mucus descriptions: MOIST ONLY; STICKY, WHITE; "; MOIST, WHITE; STICKY, "; WET, CLOUDY; TRANSP. SPINN; SLIPPERY, TRANSP.; STICKY, WHITE; THICK, "; "

Fig 5.3 Interrupted mucus pattern as a result of stress
Note: Any days which become dry after one or more days of mucus should be considered fertile.

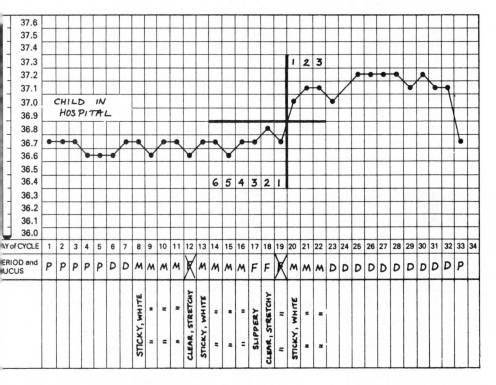

Fig 5.4 Double peak caused by stress

function in varying degrees, resulting in either a delayed ovulation or the complete suppression of ovulation.

If the stress occurs during the pre-ovulatory phase, then the mucus pattern may be interrupted. There may be a return to dryness as in figure 5.3. Ovulation will be delayed either until the stress is over or the body adapts to it. Ovarian function will then return to normal and the mucus pattern will show the characteristic build-up to peak.

Some women may experience double peaks when under stress. This is seen as a build-up to peak day followed by a return to dryness or sticky mucus days, then a further episode of clear stretchy mucus several days later. If a double peak occurs, the temperature shift will be delayed until after the second peak has been observed confirming that ovulation has passed, as illustrated in figure 5.4. To avoid making errors in chart interpretation, it is vital to correlate temperature readings with mucus changes. Surprise pregnancies have occurred when couples tire of waiting for the temperature shift and presume a cycle to be infertile.

If the effect of the stress is strong enough, ovulation will be completely suppressed. The basic infertile pattern may be one of dryness throughout, or of unchanging mucus characteristics. There may be mucus changes associated with fluctuating hormone levels, but the temperature will remain on one level until the next period, resulting in an anovulatory cycle (see page 40). Ovulation may be delayed by stress for many months in extreme circumstances, for example when there has been severe weight loss as in anorexia nervosa.

THE EFFECT OF DRUGS AND DISEASES ON THE MENSTRUAL CYCLE

There is relatively little documented about the effect of drugs and diseases on the menstrual cycle. A woman should be particularly vigilant during a time of illness or stress, or when taking any form of medication. Any disturbance should be recorded on the fertility chart.

Some drugs will affect the menstrual cycle and cause irregularities in the cycle length, the mucus pattern or the temperature. If drugs are prescribed to treat infections, the disturbance may be caused as much by the infection and the stress it imposes on the body as by the medication. Any infection is likely to be accompanied by a pyrexia (fever) thus disturbing the temperature pattern.

Some analgesics (pain killers) such as Aspirin and paracetamol also act to reduce pyrexia. These drugs may therefore produce a lower than normal temperature reading.

The cervical mucus pattern may also be disturbed by antibiotics, because some women may develop a monilial infection or thrush due to the alteration of the normal vaginal medium.

Antihistamine drugs dry up excessive secretions from mucus membranes. As the cervix is lined by mucus membrane, the drying effect will disrupt cervical secretion. The production of cervical mucus may also be impaired by anti-inflammatory drugs such as those used in the treatment of rheumatism.

Oestrogen and progestogen therapy, which may be used in the treatment of gynaecological disorders, may affect the quality and quantity of mucus. These hormones, which are similar to those used in the contraceptive pill, may be stored in the body fat, hence their effect may be prolonged after the therapy is discontinued.

Some medications used to treat migraine, nausea, and vomiting and travel sickness; chemotherapy, powerful drugs used in the treatment of cancer, and cortisone may also cause irregularities in the menstrual cycle.

This is not considered an exhaustive list, and it should be emphasised that any stressful situation including illness or medication may cause a disturbance in the menstrual cycle and so affect the sympto-thermal chart.

MINOR DISORDERS WHICH MAY AFFECT THE CERVICAL MUCUS PATTERN

Cervical erosion or Ectropian

A cervical erosion occurs when the lining of the cervical canal grows over the lip of the cervix. When seen through a speculum it appears as a red-raw area on the cervix, which is normally pinkish-coloured. There is an increased incidence of cervical erosion as a response to oestrogen following childbirth, and also as a side effect of the contraceptive pill.

The cells of the erosion may produce a continuous discharge. With experience a woman will generally learn to distinguish this from her fertile mucus pattern. The erosion may cause a characteristic unchanging mucus pattern throughout the cycle and the onset and build-up of fertile mucus will be recognised as being significantly different and changing. If the discharge is excessive, it may cause a problem, and the affected area can be treated using cryosurgery (freezing), or laser therapy. Following such treatment, there may be a heavy, thick discharge for about two weeks, before the number of mucus days returns to normal. In most women, the cervical erosion causes no symptoms and is best left alone.

Fertility awareness in coil users

Some women who are changing from the coil (the intra-uterine contraceptive device) to natural family planning may decide to keep their
device in place during the learning period to give added security, until
they are confident in determining their fertility. The mucus pattern may
be affected.

Fertility awareness enables a woman to be more in tune with her
body's natural changes. She will be very quickly alerted to any alteration
in her normal pattern, and will thus be in a position to seek earlier
medical advice.

Fertility awareness following a dilatation and curettage (D&C)

After a dilatation and curettage, there may be a variable amount of
bleeding from slight spotting to that of a normal period, lasting from 2–10
days. There may be an interrupted mucus pattern, delayed ovulation and
a long cycle. Consequently the first normal period is frequently heavier
than normal. After this time the cycle will usually be back to normal.

6 The Cervix

CHANGES IN THE CERVIX

To use the sympto-thermal method of family planning effectively, it is not essential to check the cervix directly. The temperature and mucus observations give a woman adequate information about her state of fertility. However, some women find that monitoring changes directly at the cervix gives additional supportive information. In special circumstances, such as during breastfeeding and the pre-menopause, it can give valuable early warning signs of approaching fertility.

Changes in the cervix are due to the effect of the hormones oestrogen and progesterone. Early and late in the menstrual cycle, at the times of infertility, the cervix is low in the vagina, and easily within reach of the fingertip. It appears to be long and may be off-centre, ie tilted, to lie against the vaginal wall. It will feel firm, like the tip of a nose. The cervical opening (os) will be closed, giving the sensation of a dimple to the touch, and it will feel dry.

As ovulation approaches, the rising oestrogen levels cause the cervix to rise higher in the vagina. It appears shorter, straighter and more centrally positioned in the vagina. It may be difficult to reach. It will feel softer, more like the texture of the lower lip. The cervix relaxes slightly allowing the os to open enough to admit the finger-tip. It will feel wet and flowing with mucus.

The subtle changes in level, position, consistency and dilatation of the cervix occur gradually and may seem confusing at first, but with experience a woman will be able to recognise at least one of the characteristics which will give clear indication of her state of fertility.

To summarise:
A low, long, tilted, firm, closed, dry cervix is infertile.
A high, short, straight, soft, open, wet cervix is fertile.

The changes in the cervix take place over a period of around ten days. Approximately six to eight days before the shift in temperature the cervix . will begin to show fertile characteristics. Following ovulation, the cervix returns to its infertile state within 24–48 hours.

To avoid pregnancy, abstinence should be observed from the onset of fertile signs until the third evening of the post-ovulatory infertile cervix. Cervical signs alone should not be relied upon as a means of determining fertility.

SELF-EXAMINATION OF THE CERVIX

The cervix should be examined at the same time each day, for example while washing in the morning, after emptying the bladder.

The same position should be used to examine the cervix each day; either standing with one leg raised (eg on the side of bath), or squatting. If the position is varied, then the cervix will appear to be at a different level.

Before feeling internally for the cervix, the hands should be washed and dried (the fingernails should be short). The right index finger is gently inserted into the vagina until the cervix is palpable. It will feel like a smooth indented ball. The vaginal walls feel soft, moist and ridged in comparison. A woman can detect changes in the cervix by feeling gently with the fingertip. A delicate touch is all that is required to distinguish the subtle day-to-day changes.

If the cervix is difficult to reach, the uterus may be pushed down by pressing on the abdomen with the left hand, just above the pubic bone. With experience the whole examination should only take a few seconds.

It should be remembered that the vaginal walls are always moist, so the examining fingers will feel a bit wet. This may seem confusing at first, but women should not be discouraged. It generally takes several cycles for the changes to be interpreted accurately.

Detection of mucus at the cervix
Some mucus may come away on the finger when the cervix is checked. This may be recorded on the chart separately.

If a woman is unable to distinguish changes in sensation at the vulva, or is experiencing difficulty in defining her mucus externally, it may be helpful to take mucus directly from the cervix in this way.

An interval of a day or two may occur before thick, sticky mucus noted at the cervix is visible externally. The more liquid, fertile mucus appears at the vulva within hours. Some women may find that mucus becomes trapped in the ridged vaginal walls, and this mucus may appear as a long thread on the finger.

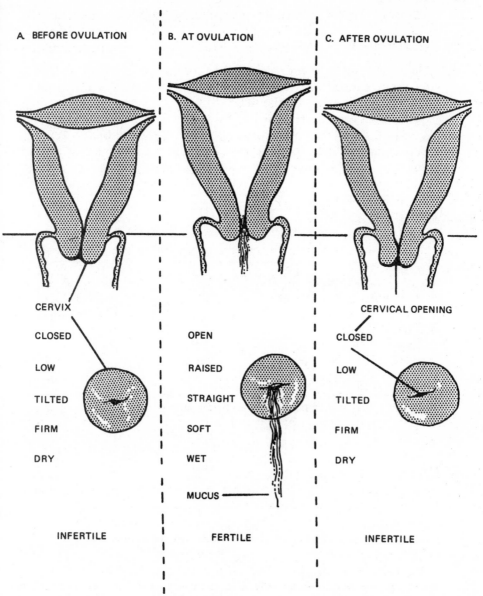

A. BEFORE OVULATION

B. AT OVULATION

C. AFTER OVULATION

CERVIX

CERVICAL OPENING

CLOSED	OPEN	CLOSED
LOW	RAISED	LOW
TILTED	STRAIGHT	TILTED
FIRM	SOFT	FIRM
DRY	WET	DRY

MUCUS

INFERTILE

FERTILE

INFERTILE

Fig 6.1 Changes in the cervix in relation to ovulation

RECORDING CERVICAL CHANGES ON THE CHART

The infertile cervix is represented by a solid black circle drawn towards the lower end of the space to show that it is low, firm and closed. A slanted line below shows the tilt.

The fertile cervix is represented by an open circle to show softness, an inner ring shows the cervix to be open. A straight line below shows the cervix straight in position. The raised level of the fertile cervix is represented by the appropriate symbol being placed higher in the space.

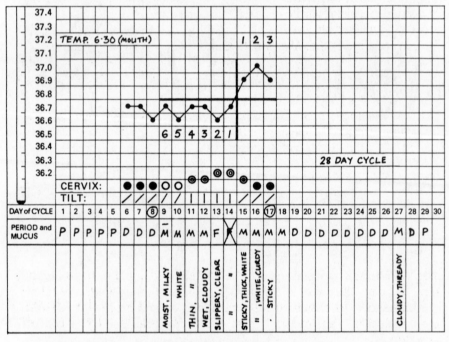

Fig 6.2 Correlation between the temperature mucus and cervical signs

Mucus first appeared on day 9, hence the last intercourse was on day 8, and was then not resumed until day 17, when the late infertile phase was confirmed:

(a) Following the third consecutive undisturbed high temperature past peak day.

(b) After the cervix had returned to its infertile state – low, firm, closed and tilted.

Cervical signs may be helpful in determining fertility, along with observation of mucus, especially at times when the temperature cannot be considered a reliable guide, such as during illness. In such circumstances intercourse should not be resumed until the fourth evening after peak day, which usually corresponds with the third evening of an infertile cervix.

Many experienced users limit their observations to the necessary part of the cycle – from the end of the period (unless a woman has a history of very short cycles), until post-ovulatory infertility is confirmed.

7 The Calendar Method and the Use of Formulae

The Calendar method – also known as the Rhythm method – is still used in a number of less developed countries. It was the first natural method, developed around 1930 when it was discovered by 'Knaus' in Austria and 'Ogino' in Japan that ovulation occurs 12–16 days before the following menstrual period regardless of the overall length of the cycle. From a record of at least six cycles the lengths of the shortest cycle and the longest cycle are noted. Allowing three days for the viability of the sperm in the female genital tract and two days for the life of the ovum and taking into account that ovulation might occur on any of 5 days in each cycle a formula was evolved:

Shortest cycle length (S) minus 20 = Last infertile day of the pre-ovulatory phase
Longest cycle length (L) minus 10 = Last fertile day

For example:-
Length of cycles during last six months = 28, 29, 28, 27, 30, 28

$S = 27$ S – 20 = Last infertile day $27 - 20 = 7$

$L = 30$ L – 10 = Last fertile day $30 - 10 = 20$

The last infertile day according to the formula is day 7 and the last fertile day is day 20. To avoid conception, couples were therefore recommended to abstain from sexual intercourse, from the 8th–20th days inclusive. This method gives an unnecessarily long period of abstinence.

It is now known that the ovum can be fertilised only within a few hours of ovulation and the viability of the sperm in the genital tract is variable and may be longer than three days. Although the calendar method is not sufficiently reliable to be recommended, nevertheless the information gained by recording the length of cycles and their variability is useful.

Detecting the early infertile phase by a formula
The formula shortest cycle minus 20 can be used to back up the mucus symptom in identifying the last day of the pre-ovulatory infertile phase.

The Doering rule

The Doering rule gives a slightly more accurate estimation of the onset of the fertile phase of the cycle. It is based on calculations made from the day of the temperature shift, which generally follows within 24 hours of ovulation.

Earliest shift day minus 7 = first fertile day

Of the previous six cycles (twelve cycles if available) identify the earliest day of the temperature rise or shift, then subtract seven days from this to give the first fertile day.

For example, if the last six cycles had temperature shifts on days 15, 16, 16, 17, 15, and 16 respectively:

$$\text{Earliest temperature rise} = \text{Day 15}$$
$$15 - 7 = 8$$
$$\text{Therefore Day 8} = \text{First fertile day.}$$

8 Minor Indicators of Fertility

OTHER PHYSICAL AND EMOTIONAL CHANGES DURING THE MENSTRUAL CYCLE

Hormonal fluctuations around the time of ovulation cause both physical and emotional changes in a woman's body. Signs may vary from one cycle to another, and different women will experience different signs, but each woman can learn to recognise those signals which will increase her awareness of fertility.

Abdominal cramps – ovulation pain (also called the Mittelschmerz symptom)

Many women will experience a short-lived stabbing pain, or dull ache on one side of the lower abdomen lasting from a few hours up to a day or so. The cause of the pain has been disputed. It may be due to contractions of the fallopian tube, or it may occur as the egg is released from the ovary. The pain may occur before, during or after ovulation.

Spotting or light bleeding

This may be caused by the effect of high oestrogen levels on the endometrium. The spotting may appear by itself, or it may tinge the fertile mucus a red/brown colour. Spotting is not a frequent occurrence, but is more common in women who experience long cycles. Spotting will occur while the temperature is still in the low phase (pre-ovulatory), or as the temperature shift is occurring. It cannot therefore be confused with true menstruation which occurs at the end of the high temperature level. **Any woman who has bleeding or spotting between periods should report this to her doctor and ensure she has regular cervical smears.**

Abdominal bloating and pressure at the vulva or rectum

Bloating of the abdomen or a feeling of pressure or fullness at the vulva or rectum may be noticed. This is caused by increased fluid retention due to the high oestrogen levels.

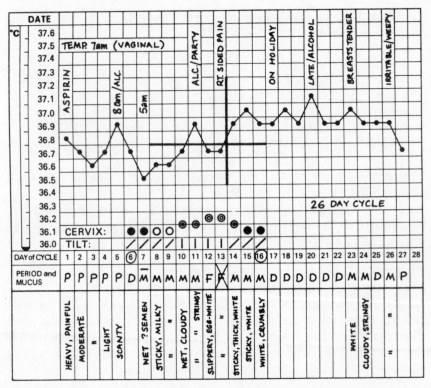

Fig 8.1 Sympto-thermal chart showing signs of bodily awareness and factors which may affect the cycle

Increased libido (sexual desire)

All women have a low level of male hormones (androgens) including testosterone in the blood. Around the time of ovulation there may be an increase in these hormones, the function being to suppress the activity of the ovarian follicles. In some women the hormonal effect may increase the libido – nature's way of encouraging sexual activity at the time most likely to achieve pregnancy. Although this phenomenon is probably related to increased androgen and oestrogen activity, it is not a universal experience.

Post-ovulatory breast tenderness and fullness

There may be slight pain, tension or tenderness in the breasts, as increasing levels of progesterone following ovulation cause the breasts to become fuller. This will often become more marked pre-menstrually, and disappear with the onset of the period.

Additional signs which may indicate fertility

There are a multitude of other signs that may be noticed including tiredness, sleeplessness, irritability, increase in energy, increase in appetite, better memory, heaviness in the legs, distinct vaginal odour, slight diarrhoea or constipation, changes in the oiliness of hair and skin, changes in complexion, pimples on the face and back or worsening of acne.

It is common for a woman to experience only some of these indicators of fertility. After a period of self-observation, a woman can identify the way her body reacts both physically and emotionally to the hormonal fluctuations in her menstrual cycle.

Pre-menstrual syndrome

Pre-menstrual syndrome is the term used for a collection of symptoms which occur one to two weeks before a menstrual period (post-ovulatory phase). The symptoms disappear at the onset of menstruation. Pre-menstrual syndrome should not be confused with dysmenorrhoea (painful periods), the symptoms of which appear the day before or at the onset of menstruation and disappear at its end.

Symptoms of pre-menstrual syndrome (often known as pre-menstrual tension or PMT) include irritability, nervous tension, moodswings, crying, depression, headache, loss of energy, breast tenderness, abdominal bloating, weight gain and craving for sweets, especially chocolate. The severity of the symptoms may vary from a nuisance value in mild cases, to causing serious disruption of family and social life in severely affected women.

LORNA: Depression. The very word makes people feel low. Lorna suffered from severe bouts of depression, hard on her husband, bad for Jean and Tim her children and rotten for herself. Sometimes she felt she was going mad.

Keeping charts really helped Lorna. She charted her temperature and mucus signs and she also recorded her emotions, good days and days when she felt depressed. There on the chart, as clear as daylight, she could see that her bad days were related to her cycle. Depression started a week before her period, sometimes earlier but always ceased within 48 hours of the beginning of the period. She knew it was physical, and not 'all in the mind'. Lorna went back to her doctor, who recommended hormone treatment, which solved the problem for her and also for her family.

If a woman is disturbed by such symptoms, she should consult her doctor. Pre-menstrual syndrome may be associated with low levels of progesterone in the post-ovulatory phase. Progesterone therapy may be most effective for these women. Supplements of pyridoxine or vitamin B6 have also proved beneficial for some women. Some doctors are now looking at dietary habits and stressing the advantage of natural foods and restricting highly refined foods, sugar and stimulants such as tea, coffee and alcohol.

9 Planning a Family by the Sympto-Thermal Method

TO CONCEIVE

When a couple are planning a pregnancy, knowledge of their combined fertility will help to determine the time of conception.

Timing of intercourse for the couple desiring pregnancy

The most favourable time for conception is the last day of the fertility symptoms, peak day, when there is a wet, lubricative sensation at the vulva, the presence of thin, transparent stretchy mucus, like raw egg white; and when the cervix is high, straight, soft, open and flowing with fertile mucus. These conditions are normally found on the day of ovulation or the day preceding ovulation. The temperature rise may be expected to occur one to two days later. Conception is possible at any time during the defined fertile period.

A couple who have not achieved pregnancy after one year (following regular intercourse at the fertile time of the cycle), should see their general practitioner who may advise further investigations of infertility.

Early *miscarriage* is common. If the temperature stays high for more than twenty days and is then followed by a fall and a heavy painful period with clots, this usually indicates a very early miscarriage. This is nature's way of handling the abnormal conception, but if it is a recurring problem, it may be due to immunological factors. Following a miscarriage, charting should be continued. Cycles usually return to normal fairly quickly.

PRE-CONCEPTUAL CARE

When a couple are planning a pregnancy there are many advantages to improving good general health in the pre-conceptual period, to provide optimum conditions for conception, pregnancy, birth and subsequent childcare.

Both partners should enjoy a well-balanced diet, avoiding excessive amounts of fatty foods or sugars, and eating plenty of fresh fruit, whole

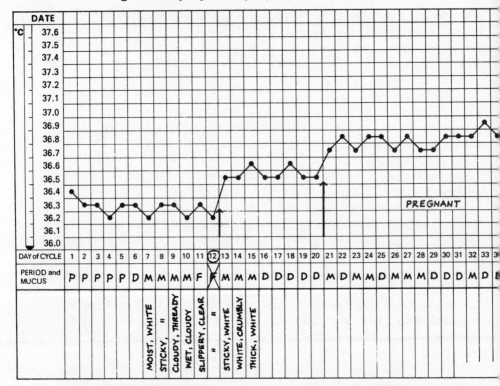

Fig 9.1 Achieving pregnancy
The couple aimed to conceive. Intercourse on day 12 in the presence of fertile mucus was followed by a shift in temperature the following day. Conception had taken place.

In cycles where conception occurs many women will record a second increase in temperature to an even higher level, several days after the ovulation shift. Note further temperature elevation on day 21. This is due to increased production of progesterone which occurs as implantation takes place.

If pregnancy is established, there is no fall in temperature at the time of the next expected menstruation. A post-ovulatory high temperature lasting more than twenty days indicates a probable pregnancy. This is the earliest available evidence of pregnancy. A pregnancy test should be done to confirm it.

grain foods, and vegetables. Maintenance of an optimum weight for height is important. Any woman who is either very underweight or overweight may have difficulties in conceiving. Alcohol should be reduced to a minimum or given up, as in excess it can seriously affect the developing foetus. Smoking should likewise be stopped prior to conception because it reduces the oxygen supply to the developing foetus and may result in a baby of low birth weight and poor health. The incidence of miscarriages is also significantly higher in women who smoke. It is a wise precaution to avoid all drugs in the pre-conception period and during pregnancy and breastfeeding. The only medications that should be taken are those prescribed by a doctor who is aware of the pregnancy or impending conception. Adequate rest and sleep are important. Undue fatigue and stress should be avoided. It may be a good time to learn a relaxation technique that will be beneficial during pregnancy, childbirth and in the later years. Moderate amounts of daily exercise are important to promote a sense of well-being and maintain fitness (but not excessive fanatical exercising which may cause weight loss, hormone imbalance and anovulation).

It is important that a couple enjoy sex and do not become too pre-occupied with plans for conception. If sex is pleasurable for both partners, then it is likely to be more frequent and the relationship will be enhanced.

Whenever possible a couple should discuss with their doctor their intentions to plan a pregnancy. The opportunity may arise naturally if a method of contraception is stopped in order to achieve pregnancy, for example if a coil is removed. But by the nature of natural family planning, there may be no such apparent opportunity for discussion with a doctor. The most essential aspect of pre-conceptual care is to ensure that a woman is immune to rubella (German measles). If the developing foetus is exposed to the rubella virus in the first twelve weeks, there may be catastrophic effects including blindness, deafness and mental retardation. This can be avoided by a simple blood test to detect rubella antibodies in the mother's blood.

SEX DETERMINATION

The sex of a child is determined by the father at the time of conception, when either an X chromosome or a Y chromosome sperm fertilises the ovum to produce a girl or a boy respectively.

According to the work of Dr Shettles, an American gynaecologist, the timing of intercourse in relation to the quality of cervical mucus is a crucial factor in sex determination. Around the time of ovulation the alkaline peak mucus provides the optimum conditions for sperm survival of both types of sperm.

The Y sperm are lighter than the X sperm, and able to move more rapidly towards the ovum, so the chances of a boy are increased by a single act of intercourse on peak day or the day following peak, as close as possible to the predicted ovulation.

A single act of intercourse two to three days before ovulation, when fertile mucus signs are just beginning, at the transition from thick, cloudy mucus to thin, transparent mucus increases the chances of a girl. The less alkaline medium of early transition mucus favours the survival of the more acid-resistant X chromosome sperms.

Extensive, reliable studies are not available to support this theory, and at least thirty other variables that may influence sex have been reported, such as the rising female birthrate with increasing parental age and an increasing male birthrate with higher socio-economic status, and frequency of intercourse.

Books and magazine articles about the timing of intercourse and the effect of acid or alkaline douching have brought the subject of sex determination to the public eye. Couples have nothing to lose by testing out this theory, but they should be aware of the realistic chances. The percentage change in sex ratio achieved by these measures is probably only altered by around 5–10 per cent, and 50 per cent of the couples will achieve the sex of their choice anyway.

Possibility of birth defects

It is periodically suggested that there may be an increased risk of birth defects and miscarriages in NFP users because a high proportion of unplanned pregnancies will result from intercourse at the outer limits of fertility when the sperm or the ovum are aged. The evidence to support this theory results from animal experiments using aged sperm and ova. At present, there is no evidence to suggest an increased incidence of either birth defects or miscarriages in humans under these circumstances.

In a large WHO Multicentre Trial of the ovulation method, researchers looked at the outcome of 160 pregnancies. They found that the spontaneous abortion rate was 10 per cent lower than the 25 per cent for the general population and the rate of congenital malformation was 1.25 per cent, the same as that for the general population. The study concluded that spontaneous abortions (miscarriages) and congenital malformations or birth defects were not related to the time-interval between sexual intercourse and ovulation.

Couples practising natural family planning have the advantage that the method does not involve the introduction of drugs, chemicals or irritants into the body, so a naturally occurring pregnancy will not be affected by any of these potential hazards.

TO AVOID PREGNANCY

Identification of the pre-ovulatory infertile phase
The pre-ovulatory infertile phase may be identified by the mucus symptom, cervical signs, a calendar calculation or the Doering rule.

By the mucus symptom
Following the period, dry days are infertile.

It is wise to use alternate evenings for intercourse, because the presence of seminal fluid in the vagina may mask cervical mucus.

The day on which cervical mucus is first recognised marks the end of this phase.

By cervical signs
For those women who wish to use the additional information given by changes in the cervix, the following rules apply:-

From the end of the period, days on which the cervix is low, firm, closed and tilted are infertile. The first day of change in position or texture marks the end of this phase.

By calculation
Calculations made by calendar or the Doering rule should be worked out on evidence given by recording information from at least six cycles, and preferably from twelve cycles.

Calendar calculation
The shortest cycle minus twenty gives the last infertile day. The pre-ovulatory infertile phase lasts from the first day of the cycle until the last infertile day inclusive.

The Doering rule
The earliest day in the cycle on which the temperature shift has been seen to occur minus seven gives the first fertile day. The pre-ovulatory infertile phase lasts from the first day of the cycle up to, but not including the first fertile day.

By the sympto-thermal method
The information given by the above observations should be considered together and the *earliest indication* of the end of the infertile phase should be accepted.

Effectiveness of the pre-ovulatory infertile phase
Intercourse in the pre-ovulatory infertile phase always carries a slight risk of pregnancy. It is in this phase we consider male fertility, because in the presence of early mucus, the life of the sperm may be prolonged.

In some cases ovulation could occur earlier than anticipated, but an experienced woman will be alerted to changes in sensation and will be forewarned of an early ovulation provided she remains vigilant.

In a small minority of women, with short cycles of around 19-24 days, or with prolonged menstrual bleeding, mucus may appear immediately after the period or even before its end. In this case intercourse during a period could lead to conception. There will be no pre-ovulatory infertile phase.

Identification of the post-ovulatory infertile phase
By the sympto-thermal method
Using the double check of mucus and temperature, the post-ovulatory infertile phase starts on the morning on which the third high temperature has been recorded, provided that all three high temperatures are past peak mucus day.

Effectiveness of the post-ovulatory infertile phase
It should be emphasised that the post-ovulatory infertile phase is the safest time for intercourse for a couple wishing to avoid pregnancy.

Where there are very serious contra-indications to pregnancy, Dr Joseph Roetzer's 'life or death' rules may be adopted. Intercourse should be restricted to the post-ovulatory completely infertile time, by waiting until the evening of the fourth day of higher temperature readings before assuming infertility.

If the mucus pattern is not recognised, Dr Roetzer advises that infertility should not be assumed until the evening of the fifth day of higher temperatures to avoid any misinterpretation of the temperature shift. These 'life or death rules' are as reliable as male or female sterilisation.

KATE AND QUENTIN: Kate attended an interest talk on NFP hoping to learn where she had gone wrong. She and Quentin had not intended to start a family, not yet. She had read the Billings book and from that had taught herself to observe the mucus signs. She had obeyed the rules, so why was she pregnant?

Kate was interested to learn about the sympto-thermal method and at the end of the talk, she arranged an appointment for herself and Quentin to see one of the teachers in NFP. She took her charts with her and it was clear that observation of mucus only two days before 'peak' gave insufficient warning of approaching ovulation. Since the birth of their baby, Kate and Quentin have had no problems in using a natural method of family planning. Using the Doering rule to identify the end of the pre-ovulatory, infertile phase, the mucus signs and the temperature chart to identify the beginning of the post-ovulatory phase, they have found the method reliable. Their second child was planned and conception occurred as expected.

Why various organisations use different rules

During the last twenty years, programmes for teaching natural family planning have been implemented in more than ninety countries throughout the world. Various organisations have been concerned in this work. Each organisation has produced its own charts and teaching material and has developed its own guidelines for identifying the fertile and infertile phases of the cycle. These guidelines reflect the emphasis laid on efficiency and acceptability for peoples of different cultures.

The number of days of abstinence will vary according to the flexibility of the rules. Some organisations will sacrifice a certain degree of efficiency to allow a method which is culturally and practically acceptable. In India, the modified mucus method is used extensively as it is felt necessary to reduce the time of abstinence in order to obtain a wider number of users. Abstinence is limited to the days of slippery stretchy mucus and two days and nights after peak mucus day.

The Billings method allows intercourse on the evenings of alternate dry days in the pre-ovulatory infertile phase and unrestricted intercourse in the post-ovulatory infertile phase from the fourth day after peak mucus symptom. Intercourse must be avoided during menstruation.

The Hilgers ovulation method has similar rules to Billings but uses a special mucus scoring system. Women wishing to learn the Hilgers method must be instructed by Hilgers trained teachers.

How the length of abstinence varies according to the chosen rules

Fig 9.2 shows the approximate length of abstinence and the time available for intercourse in a hypothetical 28 day cycle for a woman who has cycles ranging from 28–31 days.

Where mucus only methods are used to prevent pregnancy, the length of abstinence in the pre-ovulatory phase depends on the length of the period, the number of dry days and the type of mucus observed.

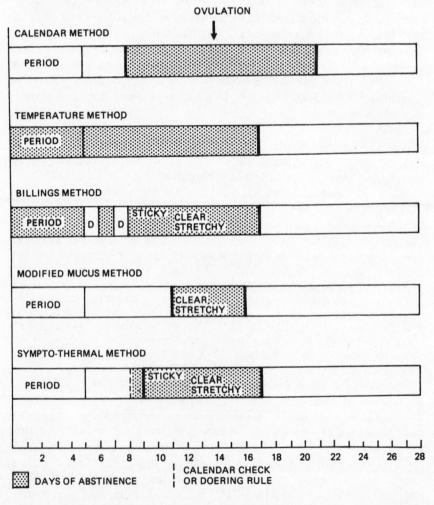

Fig 9.2 The length of abstinence required by different natural methods of family planning

The length of abstinence required by couples using the sympto-thermal method will vary according to the strictness of the rules. Some couples may require the highest degree of efficiency and will be prepared to abstain for longer periods to achieve this, whereas other couples may be in a position to relax the rules a little to allow more time for intercourse, although in doing so they will reduce the efficiency. Couples using natural family planning are able to adopt guidelines to suit their circumstances.

Fig 9.3 Advantages and disadvantages of natural methods of family planning

Advantages	*Disadvantages*
1 No physical side effects and no interference with the woman's normal physiology.	1 Relatively long initial instruction.
2 Both partners share the responsibility for planning their family. The education necessary for fertility awareness may lead to better communication and may contribute to a more co-operative relationship in other areas of marriage.	2 There may be fear of unplanned pregnancy because though method failure is low, there is a higher user failure rate particularly during the learning period.
3 Can be used to help couples achieve pregnancy.	3 There has to be an acceptance of abstinence by both partners requiring high motivation and commitment.
4 Cost-effective. After initial training the couples are independent and have control over their own fertility.	4 There may be difficulty using natural methods for some women in the times when their physiology is undergoing change; after childbirth, after taking the contraceptive pill and during the pre-menopause.
5 Women who use this method find that they are able to monitor their own health.	
6 Morally and culturally acceptable in societies where artificial contraception is unacceptable.	

10 Effectiveness

COMPARISON OF NATURAL FAMILY PLANNING WITH CONTRACEPTIVE METHODS

When considering the effectiveness of any form of birth control, the distinction must be made between the theoretical or method effectiveness (biological effectiveness) and the practical or use effectiveness. Since the 1930s the accepted measure of contraceptive effectiveness has been the pregnancy rate per 100 women-years of use, according to the Pearl Index. This shows how many women would get pregnant if 100 women used a given method of birth control for one year. The method effectiveness is the maximum effectiveness of the method when used without error or omission, that is when used according to instructions. The failure rate is known as the theoretical or method failure rate. In theory the failure rate for the sympto-thermal method, for example, is around 2 per cent.

The use effectiveness takes into consideration all users of the method, that is those who follow the method without error and also those who are careless. It denotes the effectiveness under real life conditions. The failure rate is referred to as the practical or user failure rate, for example the sympto-thermal method has a user failure rate of 4–15 per cent.

The table opposite gives the generally accepted comparative figures for the different methods of birth control.

A couple's motivation has a crucial influence on the use effectiveness of all methods of family planning. The first year's use always carries the highest risk of unplanned pregnancy due to the time taken for a couple to adapt to the chosen method. Barrier methods require some skill and a high degree of motivation, pills are more frequently forgotten and coils are more likely to be expelled in the first year.

EFFECTIVENESS OF NATURAL FAMILY PLANNING

A high degree of motivation is essential if a couple are to use natural methods of family planning successfully. They should both be in accord about their goals of family spacing or limiting. It is interesting to note that

Fig 10.1 Comparison of failure rates of different methods of birth control

Family planning method	Theoretical or method failure	Practical or user failure
Sterilisation Male and Female	0.15	0.5–2
Injectable progestogens	0.25	1
Combined pill	0.1	1
Progestogen only pill	0.5	4
I.U.C.D.	2	5
Condom	2	3–15
Diaphragm	2	4–12
Periodic abstinence (calendar, ovulation and sympto-thermal)	2–5	10–30
Ovulation method	1–5	6–28
Sympto-thermal	1–3	4–15
Contraceptive sponge	11	15

Fig 10.2 Comparison of natural family planning failure rates in various World Health Organisation studies

Study	NFP method		Number of participants	Method failure	Overall user failure
Parenteau-Carreau, Lanctot, Rice 1976 USA	sympto-thermal		168	0.7	6.0
Analysis of above study	spacers limiters		67 101		14.9 1.1
Barbato, Bartoletti 1988 Italy	sympto-thermal		460		3.6
Clubb, Pyper, Knight 1988 UK	sympto-thermal		72		2.7
Wade 1979 USA	sympto-thermal ovulation	comparative study			9.4 24.8
Rice, Lanctot, Garcia-Devesa 1979 USA	sympto-thermal		1,022		7.5
WHO multi-centre trial 1980	ovulation		869	2.8	19.6
Marshal 1982 UK	sympto-thermal	experienced users	108	0.3	3.9

the family-spacers, those who plan more children but at a later date, are less effective in preventing pregnancy. They are prepared to take risks; whereas family limiters, those who have completed their family, are more conscientious and determined, and more successful in preventing pregnancy. This is illustrated in figure 10.2 by the 1976 American sympto-thermal study which showed a failure rate of almost 15 per cent for the family spacers and around 1 per cent for those limiting their families.

It is interesting to note that the 1979 American study comparing the sympto-thermal with the ovulation method shows the sympto-thermal method to be twice as effective, because there is less chance of making an error when there is a double check available.

The effectiveness of any form of birth control depends on the method being well taught, well understood and well applied, but this is of particular importance for natural family planning. With experience, the sympto-thermal method is a highly effective method. This is illustrated in figure 10.2 by the Marshall study of experienced users where there was an overall failure rate of 3.9 per cent. The degree of efficiency afforded by the sympto-thermal method depends on the guidelines adopted.

Effectiveness of the pre-ovulatory infertile phase

Pre-ovulatory infertile days can be effective if the pre-ovulatory calculation S minus 20 to determine the last infertile day, (or preferably the Doering Rule) is checked against the observation of the first sign of mucus.

A 1984 study, by Dr Anna Flynn, of eight experienced users of the sympto-thermal method concluded that the most reliable indicator to detect the beginning of the fertile period, was the calendar calculation, S minus 20. Mucus was not always present sufficiently early to warn of approaching fertility. One pregnancy resulted from intercourse on a dry day which was calculated by ultrasound scan and hormone assays to be five days before ovulation. If the S minus 20 rule had been applied it was reasonably assumed that the pregnancy might not have occurred as sexual intercourse would have been discontinued two days previously.

The couple who accept the very slight possibility of pregnancy may use the pre-ovulatory infertile days. Since unplanned pregnancies usually arise from intercourse in the pre-ovulatory phase and during the first two years of use of the method, the inexperienced couple should be advised not to use these days before they are confident in determining the onset of fertile signs, if there is a strong need to avoid pregnancy.

Effectiveness of the post-ovulatory infertile phase

The post-ovulatory infertile days ensure the highest degree of efficiency. Beginners in the method should use only the post-ovulatory infertile days for intercourse. It is helpful if the instructor can identify the late infertile phase with the couple for the first two or three cycles or until they feel sufficiently confident to determine this alone. Adding a day or two to allow for misinterpretation of the peak day will increase the rate of success in the learning period.

In the 1982 Marshall study which included women with normal fertile cycles and women in special circumstances, where the overall failure rate was 3.9 per cent, there were no pregnancies resulting from intercourse after the third high temperature was recorded.

Dr Joseph Roetzer considers the reliability of his 'life and death' rule to be comparable to that for male or female sterilisation (see p 74).

Effectiveness of teaching NFP in general practice

A community-based project was carried out in a NHS health centre in Oxford, to assess the efficiency and cost-effectiveness of teaching the sympto-thermal method. A practice nurse used group teaching and audio-visual aids (Fig 10.2) Seventy-two women wishing to avoid pregnancy charted 903 cycles with an overall failure rate of 2.7 on the Pearl Index. In this study there were 26 couples with fertility problems wishing to conceive; 19 were successful.

The cost per patient based on five hours teaching was £27.90. This compared favourably with other methods of contraception (See Fig 10.3).

Figure 10.3 Comparative cost with other methods of contraception over two years

Hormonal contraception	£46.90
Intra-uterine contraceptive device	£69.40
Diaphragm and spermicide	£51.10
Sympto-thermal method: Four hours teaching (normal fertility)	£23.50
Five hours (Special Circumstances)	£27.90

Living with natural family planning

Couples should be comfortable with their chosen method of family planning, since its effectiveness depends to some extent on its acceptability to both partners. This is particularly true for those who use a natural method.

To be fully effective, natural methods rely on a high degree of commitment from both partners to adjust to the naturally occurring cycles of fertility and infertility. Many couples who use natural methods find their communication improves and their sexual relationship is enhanced as they discover ways to express their feelings for each other at times when intercourse is not possible.

The subject of living with natural family planning is discussed more fully on p 170.

Special Circumstances

11 Natural Family Planning Following Childbirth

BREASTFEEDING AND ITS EFFECTS ON FERTILITY_____

Breastfeeding is the natural way to space a family. Amongst the peoples of developing countries, there is far more effective family planning from breastfeeding than from all other methods of artificial contraception. The World Health Organisation has been alarmed by the rapid increase in population in countries where artificial (bottle) feeding has been introduced.

Research studies have been carried out which are of particular significance among the Eskimos and among the rural Indians of North America. In these cultures, no other form of contraception was being used and there was no taboo on sexual intercourse during lactation. The time taken for 50 per cent of the women to conceive again was 6 months in those artificially feeding but an average of 18–24 months among the breast-feeders.

Among the Kung hunter-gatherers of the Kalahari desert who have no alternatives to prolonged breastfeeding, the average time between births is 3–4 years and the average family size is 4.4 children. In view of this evidence, World Health Organisation recommends that breastfeeding should be maintained in areas of the world where mothers are able and willing to nurse their babies. In its educational programmes, WHO teaches that breast milk is the perfect food for the baby. It provides all the nutrients, the composition of breast milk changing daily during the early weeks to suit the needs of the growing infant. In addition breast milk contains the antibodies needed to protect the baby against infection and also protects the child from some allergies.

There are advantages to the mother in breastfeeding. Breastfeeding is good for her health and for her figure. Stimulation of the breasts by the nursing baby will cause reflex contractions of the uterus preventing prolonged blood loss and discharge and promoting a rapid return to normal physiology. During pregnancy the average weight gain is about 12 kilograms. One third of this is the energy reserve for producing breast milk. A breastfeeding mother will lose weight and so regain her figure more quickly provided she eats sensibly. Breastfeeding helps to develop the bonds of affection between mother and baby. As the newborn baby suckles, the mother's love for her baby is enhanced and within a few days, the breastfed baby will recognise his own mother and turn towards her. Total or ecological breastfeeding means that the baby is fed by his mother on breast milk alone without the addition of other milk, fruit juices or solid foods. Water may be given. Ideally the baby should remain close to his mother and receive frequent stimulation from her closeness to him as well as his comfort and all his nourishment and love. The baby will be fed on demand and will also suckle for comfort instead of having a dummy or comforter.

This frequent suckling is important to maintain infertility during lactation. It is interesting that the Kung hunter-gatherers have an unusual pattern of suckling, not 10 or 20 minutes from each breast every four hours, but for a few seconds or a couple of minutes four times an hour.

PHYSIOLOGY

Following childbirth, all women produce large amounts of the hormone prolactin, which stimulates the production of breast milk. Prolactin also acts on the ovary to inhibit the production of oestrogen. The low level of oestrogen during breastfeeding suppresses the maturation and ripening of the follicles and thus prevents ovulation. Within hours of delivery, there is an increase in the sensitivity of the nerve endings in the nipple so that each act of suckling stimulates the secretion of prolactin. The level falls again after 3–4 hours, but if the baby suckles frequently, including short spells of comfort suckling, the high level of prolactin is sustained thus preventing ovulation.

In 1981 Professor Howie and others carried out research on mothers to compare the return of fertility among bottle feeders and breastfeeders. The mothers who were bottle feeding had all resumed ovulation and menstruation by fifteen weeks, averaging a return of fertility between 9 and 13 weeks postpartum. But among the breastfeeding mothers, he found that there was no ovulation during total breastfeeding and that ovulation and menstruation were delayed for a variable length of time during weaning.

Howie found that ovulation occurred early among those women who suckled infrequently and introduced supplements rapidly and stopped night feeds. By contrast, those in whom ovulation was delayed maintained night feeds, introduced supplements slowly and cut down the frequency and length of suckling time gradually. In the first group, ovulation occurred rapidly after weaning was started, around sixteen weeks, but in the second group, the return of fertility in some women was delayed for up to fifteen months or longer. Howie found that ovulation did not occur among breastfeeding mothers who gave at least five feeds, totalling 65 minutes a day.

Breastfeeding should be a happy experience for the mother, but too often problems arise, sore or cracked nipples, tender breasts or a fretful unsatisfied baby, and breastfeeding is abandoned in favour of the bottle. These problems are unnecessary and should never occur. Every mother needs help when she starts to breastfeed her baby.

Firstly it is important to realise that the nipple does not fill with milk like the teat on a bottle, so the baby must not suck the nipple (which causes pain and soreness), but must open his mouth wide to take in the whole of the coloured area of the areola and so draw milk from the breast through the nipple.

If the baby is properly positioned at the breast, there should be no problems. Breastfeeding will be a satisfying experience for mother and child and the parents will be able to rely on this natural time of infertility in which to resume sexual intercourse without anxiety about another pregnancy. The couple who wish to use natural family planning during this time will be taught to recognise the mother's infertility and the signs of returning fertility.

If a woman was already aware of her fertile pattern before she became pregnant, she should have little difficulty in recognising the return of her fertility, but learning the method during breastfeeding means that much patience will be needed.

JILL AND DONALD: Jill and Donald had wanted a big family, but they were happy with their four children under six and wanted to call a halt.

Spacing as far as it had happened at all was a result of breastfeeding. However, Thomas, the youngest, had weighed 10lbs at birth. Jill had developed varicose veins and her blood pressure had been raised during the last three weeks of her pregnancy. She came to learn natural methods towards the end of breastfeeding. The teacher was concerned. Here was a client who should on no account become pregnant, wanting to learn from the beginning, at a time when the signs and symptoms of fertility and infertility would be difficult to recognise.

She told Jill that 'Natural methods can not solve every problem'. Jill was adamant she wanted to use natural methods, so the teacher insisted that Donald must attend as well, even if it meant bringing all the family. The first session was a long one. Donald and Jill were glad to discuss their problems, their feelings for each other and for their family, and to explain their attitudes to marriage and family planning. They were willing to abstain for the necessary time while they learnt the method. At the next session, fitted in during the same week, Jill and Donald learnt the basis of natural methods and the rudiments of charting. Mucus recognition was a problem which continued long after Thomas was weaned. But Jill's periods had become regular, and the biphasic temperature chart allowed them to use just the post-ovulatory infertile period for intercourse.

Jill also learnt self-examination of the cervix. In the next cycle she not only found it easy to recognise the changes taking place on the chart, but for the first time she recognised the crystal-clear stretchy, fertile mucus as it appeared like a thread when she withdrew her finger. So seven months from their first visit to the NFP teacher, Jill and Donald were independent and confident in using a natural method of family planning.

RECORDING ON THE BREASTFEEDING CHART

The breastfeeding chart should be used to record as much information as possible about mother and baby. Each chart covers eight weeks.

Baby
1. The number of feeds per day and the approximate suckling time should be calculated. Extra fluids or solids should be recorded.
2. The longest interval between feeds over 24 hours should be noted.
3. A record should be kept of baby's appetite, alterations in suckling vigour, general health, including teething, immunisation etc.

Mother
1. Basal body temperature should be recorded.
2. Mucus signs (sensation, observation and finger-testing) must be recorded. Observations should be made throughout the day and recorded in the evening. Infertile, dry days are marked in green with a 'D'. Moist days forming the basic infertile pattern are marked in green – with an 'M' added. Fertile days are marked in yellow. When fertile-type mucus is present an 'F' is added. Any bleeding is marked in red.
3. The cervix may be examined each morning and changes recorded.

4. General health and any stress should be recorded, and taking alcohol or drugs should also be noted. (All medication should be prescribed by a doctor who is aware that the mother is breastfeeding.)
5. If milk is expressed to give to the baby at a later stage (for example if the mother has to leave him/her for a while), a note must be made on the chart.
6. Any change in circumstances, such as a holiday or travel should be recorded.

Breastfeeding should be a pleasurable, relaxed experience for both mother and baby.

As a woman records her breastfeeding experience and state of infertility, she will gain confidence in the knowledge of how her body is reacting to various influences from her baby, and the environment. Throughout this time intercourse should be enjoyed without any anxiety about conception.

RECOGNISING THE BASIC INFERTILE PATTERN – INFERTILITY AWARENESS

After childbirth there follows a week or so of blood-stained discharge known as the lochia. This will diminish and give way to a recognisable state of infertile mucus discharge, or dryness. The recognition of her infertility is as important to the breastfeeding mother as awareness of fertility.

Mucus signs – the basic infertile pattern
Dry days are infertile.

Moist days. A constant pattern of mucus may be experienced giving a moist sensation. Provided that this mucus is unchanging day after day for over two weeks, this can be regarded as the infertile mucus pattern. The mucus may be thin, white and milky, or there may be a slight stickiness only and a yellowish discharge. The essential thing to establish is its unchanging characteristics. Any dry days found during a pattern of constant, unchanging mucus are infertile.

Temperature
The temperature will be swinging from high to low, that is, the day-to-day variation will be greater. It may be at a different level, often lower than in a normal fertile cycle. This is characteristic of the infertility associated

with breastfeeding. A woman would be well advised to start recording her daily temperature from about eight to ten weeks following the birth. As there may be many months of infertility during total breastfeeding, some individuals may prefer to rely on mucus alone, or a combination of mucus and cervical changes. The advantages of keeping a temperature record during the breastfeeding period should be explained.

a) The swinging temperature is a sign of infertility, which many women find reassuring.

b) As her fertility returns the temperature pattern will level, and ovulation will be recognised by the temperature shift.

Cervix

The cervix will return to its normal state about twelve weeks following the birth. After this time a woman may start recording changes in the cervix. She should be aware that after the birth of a baby, particularly the first baby, the cervix will not feel exactly as it did in the pre-pregnant state. The os will not close as completely, even in its infertile state, and may admit the fingertip. Significant changes related to fertility will however be apparent (see Section 6, The Cervix).

RECOGNISING SIGNS OF APPROACHING FERTILITY⎯⎯⎯⎯⎯⎯⎯⎯⎯⎯⎯⎯⎯⎯⎯⎯⎯⎯⎯⎯⎯⎯⎯

Once the basic infertile pattern has been established, any change in the mucus pattern or cervix, could signify approaching fertility.

1. If the infertile pattern was of dry days, any change from the sensation of dryness, or any visible mucus would signify possible return of fertility. If the infertile pattern was of moist days, the pattern will change. There may be a change in sensation, to produce a wet or slippery sensation, or changes in quantity, colour or consistency of the mucus. Fertile-type patches of mucus may be noticed, without ovulation taking place. It may be regarded as an attempt at ovulation, as oestrogen levels fluctuate. As fertility approaches the mucus is likely to appear more frequently.

2. The temperature will level. A Canadian study by Dr Suzanne Parenteau-Carreau (1983) found that in a significant number of women the temperature levelled for one or more weeks before the shift. This could therefore supply a further valuable warning sign of impending ovulation in breastfeeding women.

3. Changes in the cervix may give the earliest information of approaching fertility. The cervix rises higher in the vagina, becomes straighter, softer, and opens up.

FACTORS WHICH MAY PRECIPITATE THE RETURN TO FERTILITY

1. Fertility is likely to return when breastfeeding becomes less frequent.
2. The introduction of mixed feeding. This includes extra drinks of fruit juice or artificial milk and the introduction of small amounts of solid food. Ovulation and conception are more common after a sharp decrease in suckling time and frequency. Abrupt weaning can therefore result in a rapid return of fertility.
3. When the baby first sleeps through the night (prolactin levels fall sharply).
4. Anxiety, stress or illness – either in mother or baby. Unlike menstrual cycles where stress tends to delay ovulation, during breastfeeding the effect of stress is to allow ovulation to occur earlier than it might otherwise. Prolactin is inhibited, the oestrogen levels rise and fertile cycles return much sooner.

SHORTENED POST-OVULATORY PHASE IN FIRST CYCLE AFTER CHILDBIRTH

The interval between ovulation and the first menstruation following childbirth is often shorter than usual. It may be as short as 8–10 days. Cycles in which the post-ovulatory phase is less than 9 days are infertile, as there is insufficient time for implantation.

Spotting, or light bleeding may occur due to a rise in oestrogens around the time of ovulation, so a woman should not automatically assume that the first bleeding is menstruation.

In 60 per cent of women, the first sign of fertility will be blood loss, which has not been preceded by ovulation (Anovulatory episode).

GUIDELINES FOR AVOIDING PREGNANCY DURING BREASTFEEDING

After the lochia has dried up, there are often episodes of vaginal blood loss as breastfeeding becomes established. This is quite common for up to six weeks. A couple should allow two to three weeks after the birth before resuming intercourse, or until the woman feels comfortable. This gives time for the lochia to diminish.

Timing of intercourse before ovulation

While a couple enjoy the infertility associated with breastfeeding, they should be aware that after ten weeks the guidelines for intercourse in the pre-ovulatory phase should be followed.

Abstinence should be observed on the day following intercourse, as seminal fluid present in the vagina may mask mucus signs.

When circumstances are changing, and there is a risk of returning fertility, it is wise to limit intercourse to evenings only to allow for change in the infertile pattern during the day. If the basic infertile pattern is of dry days, any mucus is potentially fertile. If it is one of unchanging mucus, any change could indicate returning fertility.

At the first sign of returning fertility, whether shown by the cervix or the mucus, intercourse should be avoided while the fertile signs last, and for three days after the basic infertile pattern has returned.

Any day of bleeding is potentially fertile, as there is a possibility of the bleeding being associated with ovulation. Intercourse should be avoided on these days and for the following three days.

Timing of intercourse after ovulation in the first fertile cycle

In the first cycle after childbirth, intercourse may be resumed after the fourth consecutive, undisturbed high temperature past peak day has been recorded. In subsequent cycles, the third high temperature rule may be resumed. The post-ovulatory phase is likely to be shorter than usual. Only the temperature chart will give certain evidence that ovulation has taken place. After confirmation of the post-ovulatory infertile phase, a couple can enjoy unrestricted intercourse day or night until the onset of the next period.

Pages 92–3

Fig 11.1 Infertile pattern during total breastfeeding. Breastfeeding chart from 12 to 19 weeks after childbirth. The baby is totally breastfed, the number of feeds is high and there are no supplements. Note the swinging temperature and the low firm closed tilted cervix. Sticky mucus patches during the basic infertile pattern of dryness are potentially fertile and are followed by the count of 3 before infertility is assured. There is no evidence of ovulation

Fig 11.2 Return of fertility during weaning. Breastfeeding chart continues from the 20th to the 27th week. Weaning started in the 24th week and the number of breastfeeds were decreased. Note the levelling of the temperature followed by the shift in the 26th week. The arrows show the earliest sign of fertility as indicated by the cervix or the mucus. Mucus is observed more frequently, then slippery clear stretchy mucus is observed shortly before ovulation. The post-ovulatory phase is shortened

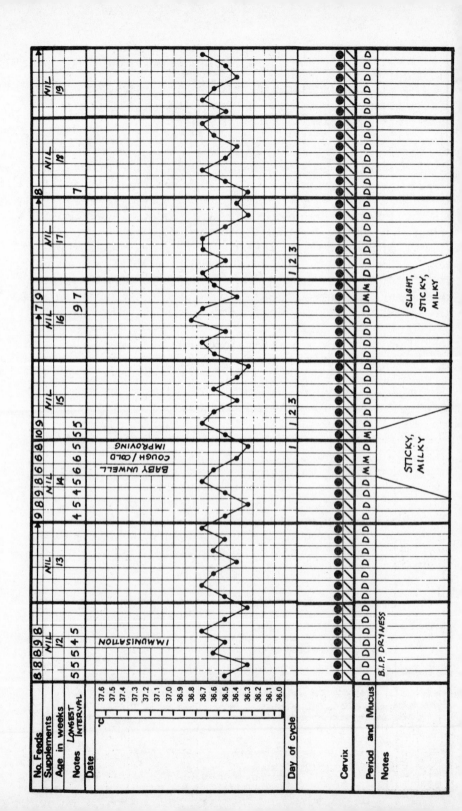

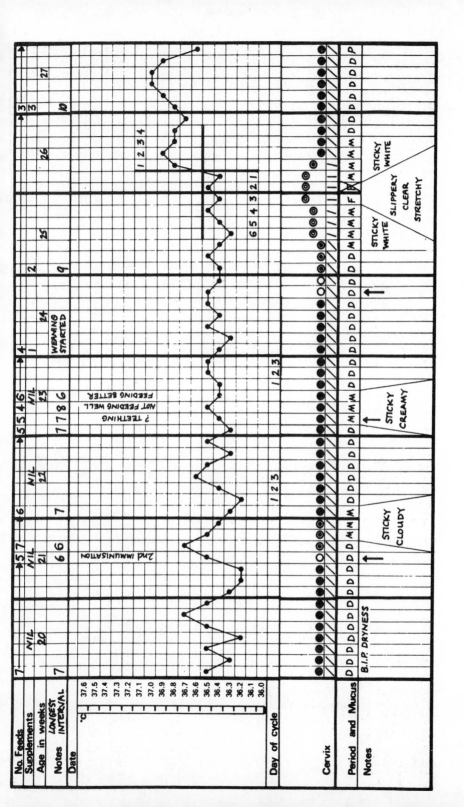

WEANING AND ITS EFFECTS ON THE RETURN OF FERTILITY———————————

If the baby is totally breastfed, weaning usually occurs in this country between four and six months. If weaning takes place gradually, this gives both mother and baby time to adjust. There may be several patches of fertile-type mucus before ovulation occurs. The pattern may seem confusing for a while. This is a time for great patience and co-operation between partners.

Fertility may return at the beginning, during, or at the end of weaning. The time taken for fertility to return, whether ovulation precedes the first menstrual period, or whether bleeding occurs with no preceding temperature shift varies from woman to woman.

Each individual breastfeeding experience in the same woman may also vary. The mucus pattern and signs indicating the onset of fertility when weaning one baby, will not automatically be the same in subsequent weaning experiences.

It is important for a woman to realise that the pattern of mucus that was infertile while she was breastfeeding may be quite changed when her menstrual cycle is back to normal, and she is no longer breastfeeding. As cycles become re-established, any pre-ovulatory mucus should be regarded as potentially fertile.

The first few cycles after breastfeeding may be of variable length. The post-ovulatory phase may be shortened (this occurs more frequently when ovulation returns within the first six months). Menstrual cycles should become more regular after a while, as hormone levels return to normal.

To apply an accurate calendar calculation as a double check for defining the onset of the fertile phase, the woman must start counting six cycles again from the start of the first menstrual period after the birth.

Lactational Amenorrhoea Method (LAM) of child spacing

LAM is based on a WHO sponsored conference, the Bellagio consensus, which concluded that a woman is 98 per cent protected from pregnancy when:

1. She is fully breastfeeding
2. The baby is less than six months old
3. Menstruation has not returned.

Promoters of LAM recognise that mucus patches may be difficult to interpret and require long periods of abstinence, which may be found unnecessary in retrospect. LAM does not require mucus observation, but simply that the above criteria are met. Any change, for example over six months post-partum, return of menses or the introduction of weaning increases the chances of pregnancy and necessitates sympto-thermal charting.

FERTILITY AWARENESS WHEN THERE IS NO BREASTFEEDING

If a woman chooses to bottle feed her baby then she may expect her fertility to return around six weeks after the birth, but ovulation may occur as early as the fourth week. In 50 per cent of women ovulation occurs before the first menstrual period. Menstruation is usual at 6–8 weeks but may be delayed to 10 weeks. The woman should start to keep her chart as soon as possible around the third or fourth week.

In the first cycle after childbirth, infertility can only be assured in the post-ovulatory phase. Intercourse may be resumed after the fourth high temperature has been recorded.

Subsequently as the mucus symptom is recognised and her normal rhythm of cycles is re-established, which may take as long as three or four months, the normal rules will apply.

FERTILITY AWARENESS WHEN THERE IS A BRIEF PERIOD OF BREASTFEEDING

If the mother breastfeeds her baby for a short time one month or less, she will be infertile for the four weeks following the birth. Ovulation may occur as early as the fifth week or may be delayed to the second or third month. Menstruation commonly occurs at the seventh or eighth week. Charting should start in the fourth week. Normal cycles are quickly re-established and the rules should be followed as before.

12 Natural Family Planning for Post Pill Users

PHYSIOLOGICAL CHANGES

The contraceptive pill causes a physiological disturbance in a woman's body. During the months after taking the pill, physiology is affected to a greater or lesser extent, possibly due to retained synthetic hormones.

Progestogen effect

The main action of the progestogen only pill in preventing pregnancy is to cause changes in the cervix keeping it hard, tightly closed and plugged with thick mucus. After discontinuing this type of pill, there is frequently considerable disturbance to the mucus pattern. This effect may also be noted due to the progestogen component of the combined pill but tends to create less of a problem.

The mucus pattern will vary from woman to woman, but most frequently there is a heavy flow of mucus for many days of the first cycle diminishing to a normal number of mucus days and a more recognisable pattern by about the third cycle. The mucus frequently shows a continual watery or milky pattern producing a wet sensation throughout. Sometimes there may be scant, sticky, crumbly mucus – either as an unchanging pattern or occurring as several patches of mucus.

Each individual's mucus pattern will be different. Mucus may be excessive and not related to the temperature shift, making it difficult to interpret the peak symptom. Rarely it may take up to six months or even longer for the woman's normal fertile pattern to return after coming off the pill.

Combined oestrogen and progestogen effect

Combined pills containing oestrogen and progestogen exert their main action in preventing ovulation. After discontinuing the combined pill, there may be a return to normal physiology very quickly, ovulation occurring within two weeks of taking the last pill, but sometimes ovulation is delayed or suppressed for a while.

Anovulatory cycles are quite common after coming off the combined pill. The temperature will stay on one level, there may be persistent dry days or an unchanging mucus pattern. In such cycles it is not possible to determine an infertile period.

There may be a combination of long, normal length and short cycles in varying sequences.

There may be several attempts at ovulation, recognisable by changes in the pattern of unchanging mucus or dryness. Oestrogen levels may rise sufficiently to cause mucus changes, but without reaching the necessary level to trigger ovulation. There may be a shortened post-ovulatory phase, around 8–10 days in some post-pill cycles.

Vaginal bleeding

Some women will complain of heavy bleeding after coming off the pill. The withdrawal bleed while taking the combined pill is generally a lighter flow, so a woman may have become accustomed to the lighter periods associated with pill use. She may also notice a change in the colour of her blood loss from a dark red/brown colour to the brighter red loss of her normal menstrual period.

Bleeding can only be recognised as true menstruation if preceded by a temperature shift approximately 14 days before. If bleeding occurs without a temperature shift in the preceding cycle, it must be regarded as a sign of potential fertility. In such circumstances, recordings should be continued on the same chart, as this is still a pre-ovulatory phase. Start a new chart at the beginning of a true menstruation.

HELEN AND TONY: Helen and Tony had used natural methods when they were first married but then on her doctor's advice Helen went on the pill.

Later on, when Helen was advised to stop taking the pill, she and Tony decided to use the sympto-thermal method again, but they ran into problems. Helen could no longer recognise her mucus. She seemed to have a continual watery or milky discharge and there were three cycles with no temperature shift. On the fourth chart there was still no shift and by the 25th day they decided (wishful thinking) that this was going to be another anovulatory cycle. They had intercourse that night. The temperature shift occurred two days later and Helen was pregnant.

This failure illustrates the problems that can arise during the months after coming off the pill.

Women should be warned of the possibility of long cycles during which ovulation may be delayed for many weeks. Unplanned pregnancies commonly occur when a couple tire of waiting for signs of fertility or the temperature shift, and assume the cycle to be anovulatory.

PILL-RELATED PROBLEMS WHICH MAY AFFECT THE MUCUS

Cervical erosion (see page 57)

If there is an excessive mucus discharge after two cycles, a woman should see her doctor. There is an increased incidence of cervical erosion caused by the effects of the pill and also following childbirth.

Candidiasis or Thrush (see page 150)

There is a higher incidence of thrush in pill users. This is generally seen as a curdy, white, irritating discharge, which can be treated quickly and effectively, usually by pessaries prescribed by the doctor.

GUIDELINES FOR AVOIDING PREGNANCY AFTER COMING OFF THE PILL

First cycle

Charting should commence as soon as possible after coming off the pill, recording the first day of the cycle from the first day of post-pill blood loss. INTERCOURSE MUST BE AVOIDED THROUGHOUT THIS CYCLE, even if there is a recognisable mucus pattern and a rise in basal body temperature.

Second cycle

INTERCOURSE MUST BE AVOIDED IN THE PRE-OVULATORY PHASE Provided there is a normal temperature shift of at least 0.2°C the post-ovulatory infertile phase can be used for intercourse, starting from the FOURTH day of the higher temperature.

Third and subsequent cycles

Intercourse should be restricted to the post-ovulatory infertile phase, until there is a recognisable mucus pattern which coincides accurately with the temperature shift. When the woman is confident that normal fertility has returned, the pre- and post-ovulatory infertile phases may be used for intercourse. The post-ovulatory infertile phase starts after the THIRD high temperature has been recorded, provided they are all past peak mucus day.

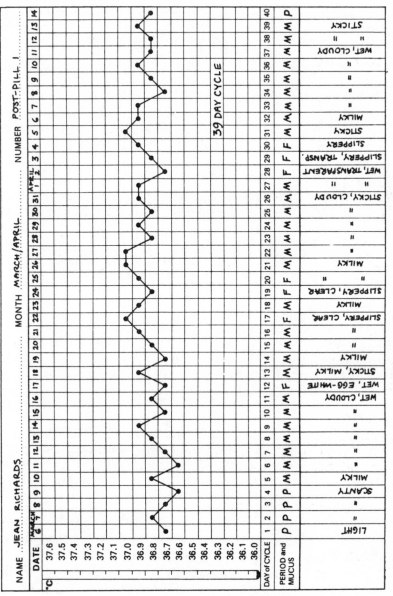

Fig 12.1 First cycle post-pill. Short period followed by a continuous pattern of milky mucus, interspersed with patches of clear stretchy mucus. Attempts at ovulation are unsuccessful and a long anovulatory cycle results. There is no recognisable infertile period

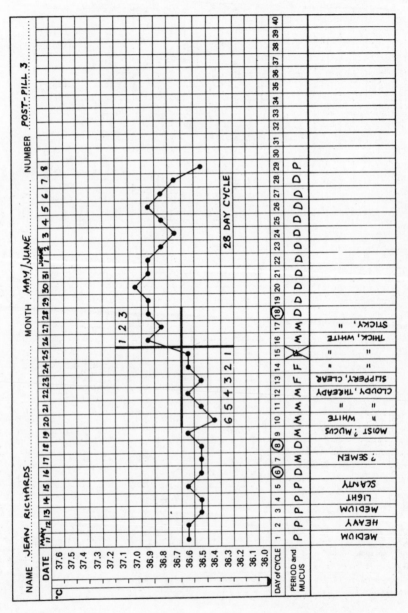

Fig 12.3 Third cycle post-pill. Recognisable mucus pattern now emerging. The post-ovulatory infertile phase begins after the third high temperature past peak day

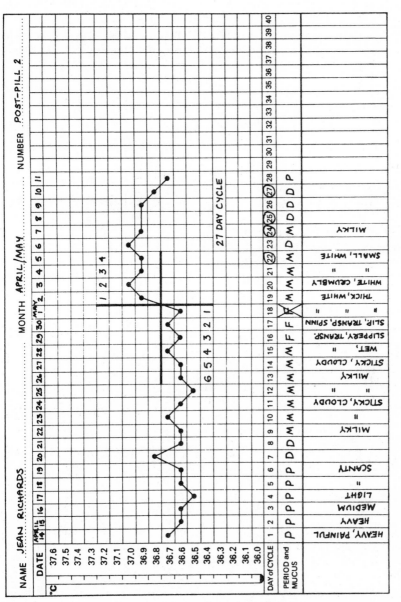

Fig 12.3 Third cycle post-pill. A normal mucus pattern coinciding with the temperature shift was observed in the previous cycle, therefore intercourse can be resumed in the pre-ovulatory phase. The post-ovulatory infertile phase begins after the third high temperature after peak day

The usual rules for using the pre-ovulatory infertile phase can be applied, if the period is shown to be a true period as confirmed by a temperature shift in the previous cycle. The calculation shortest cycle minus 20 is of no value until at least one year after discontinuing the pill.

Figs 12.1 to 12.3 illustrate return to normal fertility within three months. Remember there may be many variations as have been described.

GUIDELINES FOR CONCEIVING AFTER COMING OFF THE PILL

In the past it has been recommended that women wishing to conceive should wait for at least three cycles after stopping the pill, to allow the return of normal fertility. However, fertility clinics are now suggesting that the first three months should be used, as there may be a higher chance of conceiving during this time. In order to maximise the chances of conception, intercourse should be timed to coincide with any days on which fertile mucus is present.

Although for many women there will be little or no delay in returning fertility, Professor Vessey found in the Oxford FPA study, 1986, that impairment of fertility was greater among women over 30, particularly among those women who had never had a child. Fertility may be delayed for a year or longer, but he found no evidence suggesting that the pill causes permanent sterility.

13 Natural Family Planning During the Pre-Menopause

The last few years of a woman's fertile life are often referred to as 'the change of life'. In this country one woman in eight is experiencing the problems of this time. The natural changes are not only physical and hormonal, but there may also be psychological or emotional stress.

PSYCHOLOGICAL ASPECTS OF THE PRE-MENOPAUSE

The attitudes of society towards middle-aged women can be rather negative. There is a tendency for women to lose self-confidence and become depressed because of changes in their physical appearance, seen as signs of ageing. Ironically, a man of the same years is seen as mature and worthy of respect. Depression is counter-productive. A woman should be helped to feel self-respect. The experience of her mature years is a most valuable asset.

A positive sense of self-worth can be fostered if a woman devotes time to her own physical and mental needs. She has possibly spent the previous twenty years putting the needs of her husband and family first. As the demands on her time will inevitably decrease as her family grows up, instead of mourning this loss, she should divert her energies to meet her own needs.

Family situations may cause problems. As her children grow up they will inevitably face adolescent crises in one form or another. They may be leaving home, or embarking on marriage themselves. Emotional stress may be aggravated at this time by the ill-health or death of elderly relatives.

A woman's husband may have his own problems adapting to changing circumstances. The prospect of retirement may be a daunting one. Although men do not go through a physical or hormonal change in the way that women do, the psychological effect of the 'male menopause' cannot be denied. Communication is an essential element at every stage in a relationship, but during the 'change' partners have a particular need of each other's love, understanding and mutual support.

If a woman has a positive outlook, she can plan future activities when there will be more time for hobbies and interests. She may consider returning to some form of employment. A woman who is financially independent may have a more positive outlook on life, and the changes associated with the menopause will be minimised.

Circumstantial changes may be beyond a woman's control, but a knowledge and awareness of the body's changes can dispel fears at this time. Talking with friends who have been through, or are going through the change may help, as too will women's support groups.

PHASES OF THE MENOPAUSE

Pre-menopause
The years before menstruation ceases, when oestrogen and progesterone levels are diminishing. The lower levels of hormones are planned, and women do not suffer from a deficiency disease at this time.

Since fertility is dependent on ovulation, not menstruation, a woman over fifty years can assume permanent infertility after six consecutive anovulatory cycles. Even if she is still menstruating either regularly or irregularly, there will be no possibility of pregnancy. A woman under fifty years of age should wait for twelve consecutive anovulatory cycles, before permanent infertility is assumed.

Menopause
Ovulation and menstruation cease.

There is no further production of progesterone and a fall in oestrogen levels.

Post-menopause
There is no release or only a very minimal production of ovarian oestrogen and no further production of progesterone. Other organs such as the adrenal glands and the body fat continue to produce oestrogen, thus feminine characteristics are maintained. The levels of FSH and LH are substantially elevated in the early post-menopausal years and these high levels often reduce in later years.

PHYSIOLOGY OF THE PRE-MENOPAUSE

All female babies are born with their complement of ova (eggs) for life. No more than 390 of these cells will mature and no other ova will be formed in later life. Ova deteriorate slightly with age, hence the increased risk of chromosomal disease, such as Down's Syndrome, in babies born to older mothers. As the ovaries cease to function in mid-life, this reduces the risk of substandard eggs being fertilised.

During a woman's most fertile years, in each cycle, there are up to 30 follicles maturing in the ovary. Their combined efforts supply enough oestrogen to stimulate the process leading to ovulation.

During the pre-menopause, as a woman reaches the time when her reproductive function ceases, the ovaries produce fewer follicles. Less oestrogen is produced and attempts at ovulation are, therefore, less successful.

As the ovarian production of oestrogen decreases, the pituitary gland increases the production of FSH in an attempt to stimulate the ovaries. One of two things may happen:

1. Sometimes it succeeds; the oestrogen levels rise, the endometrium is thickened, fertile mucus is produced and ovulation occurs. Ovulation may occur early resulting in a short cycle. The period may be heavy and prolonged.
2. The follicles fail to respond. Less oestrogen is produced, the follicle will not mature and rupture, ie, no ovulation. The cycle will be long, the period short, with minimal loss.

The pattern of cycles will vary from woman to woman, and also from year to year for the same woman.

Finally the ovaries are no longer able to respond even to the increased stimulation. The hormone production will be too low to allow menstruation and ovulation. No oestrogen is produced by the ovaries after the menopause.

However, the production of oestrogen does not stop altogether after the last menstruation. The adrenal glands and body fat manufacture and store oestrogen. This is slowly released into the circulation. It may take a year or so for the adrenal glands to take over producing a baseline of oestrogen. In the meantime, the action of the male hormone, testosterone (of which small amounts are present) is unopposed by oestrogen and may contribute to feelings of irritability and aggression.

As the progesterone levels fall, the post-ovulatory phase is often shortened (8–10 days). Even if ovulation does occur, the corpus luteum is often inefficient and unable to sustain pregnancy. Eventually no more progesterone is produced.

SIGNS AND SYMPTOMS COMMONLY FOUND MENOPAUSALLY

The following list of symptoms, associated with a decrease in oestrogen levels, may sound quite alarming. Not all women will experience these symptoms sufficiently to cause any problem. If a woman is aware of the kind of symptoms to expect and understands their cause, she will see them in perspective and realise when medical advice is needed, and when symptoms are natural and should cause no anxiety.

Pre-menopausal

Menstrual irregularity For some women, menstrual periods will stop suddenly and without trouble, but the majority of women will experience some irregularity, including 'missed periods' when very long cycles occur. (See Changes that can be expected in a woman's cycle, p 110.)

Cystitis (bladder infection or inflammation) This causes frequent, painful urination. It commonly occurs among the young – hence 'honeymoon cystitis'. It may occur pre-menopausally due to slight loss of elasticity in the urinary tract tissue. Self-help measures include drinking plenty of fluids, taking mild pain-killers and resting with a hot-water bottle to ease the pain. Medical advice should be sought if symptoms persist.

Vaginitis This is a condition of dryness, soreness and irritation of the vagina and vulva which may make intercourse painful. Unhurried love-making, possibly with the use of a non-irritant lubricating cream such as KY Jelly, will help to overcome this.

Lower oestrogen levels cause thinning of the vaginal lining, making inflammation and infection more common. Vaginitis responds well to medical treatment including hormone creams.

Decline in previous ovulation signs such as bloating of the abdomen, ovulation pain, etc. The menopause may be welcomed by those women who have previously suffered from painful periods or pre-menstrual tension. If breast tenderness was a marked feature in cycles before, it may disappear altogether during the pre-menopause.

Hot flushes These are brief events caused by sudden and transient dilation of the blood vessels, during which a feeling of heat suddenly rises up the body to the head, producing redness of the neck and face and generalised perspiration which quickly subsides.

There may be – occasionally or in extreme cases – up to thirty flushes a day, then none for several weeks. Flushes may happen day or night, in severe cases causing sleep disturbance. Stress often makes flushes worse. Hot flushes are harmless and will pass. If they are slight they should be ignored. Lighter clothing, lighter bedclothes and a cooler atmosphere will help. They may cause a woman embarrassment but she should remember that other people will notice little or nothing.

Palpitations These may be experienced as the heart fluttering, or a pounding sensation in the chest. There may be transient weakness. Palpitations may accompany hot flushes or occur alone. If they are disturbing, medical advice should be sought.

Weight increase Common during the pre-menopause years. It may be exaggerated by emotional factors leading to overeating and to lack of physical exercise. If a woman becomes excessively overweight, other symptoms may be aggravated. Calorie requirements decrease with age. Although less food is needed, the diet must contain all the essential nutrients to maintain a healthy body.

A healthy diet should include sufficient fibre to give added bulk without extra calories and to maintain a regular bowel habit. Carbohydrate consumption should be low, avoiding sweet sugary foods. The diet should include plenty of fish, cheese, milk (preferably skimmed), yogurt, green vegetables, wholemeal bread and muesli.

Certain vitamin preparations are helpful in relieving symptoms such as hot flushes, tiredness and mild depression. Vitamin B6 (pyridoxine) can be taken as tablets, and may be prescribed, but pyridoxine occurs naturally in yeast, wheatgerm, bananas, chicken and meat. Vitamin E is also helpful in reducing the number and severity of hot flushes. It occurs naturally in wheatgerm and sunflower oil and can also be taken in tablet form.

Exercise, preferably outdoor, should be included as part of daily life. Exercise in any form helps increase the blood supply to the muscles, joints, and bones, to maintain fitness and encourage a sense of well-being. There is a clear relationship between a healthy body and an easier menopause.

Tiredness, insomnia, headaches, backache, nervousness, depression, memory loss and generally feeling unwell These may have a contributing physical cause.

The above-listed symptoms are transient and usually disappear around the time menstruation ceases.

A woman should attend either her general practitioner or a well-woman clinic regularly. A physical check-up will be given, including weight and blood pressure checks. A sample of urine will be tested.

Breast self-awareness is especially important during these years. Every woman should be aware of the normal shape and consistency of her breast tissue, remembering that it extends into the armpit area. During the menstrual cycle a woman's breasts naturally fluctuate in size and sometimes in tenderness. Any lumps or unusual symptoms which persist should be reported to a doctor or practice nurse. Women should be aware that breast cancer can develop at any time and early diagnosis is of vital importance.

A woman should have a cervical smear test regularly or as advised by the doctor. This simple test is used to detect early changes that occur in the cervix before cancer develops. If abnormal cells are found, cancer may be prevented.

Post-menopausal signs and symptoms

Osteoporosis is a condition caused by a decrease in oestrogen levels, where the bones become more brittle due to lack of calcium – hence the significantly higher incidence of fractures in women over 50 and later in life.

A diet rich in calcium and vitamin D is essential to maintain bone density. Milk, cheese and yogurt are rich sources of calcium. Vitamin D is found in butter, fish, meat and sunlight. In addition to a healthy diet, regular exercise is important to aid circulation to muscles, joints and bones to prevent symptoms of rheumatism, and development of the 'dowager's hump' later in life.

Skin changes – some drying and wrinkling may occur. Attention to diet, general good health, regular exercise, relaxation and use of skin preparations will help to maintain skin texture. Smoking and heavy drinking should be discouraged.

Breast changes, including some shrinkage of breast tissue. A well-fitting bra will give support.

Shrinkage of vaginal and vulval tissue, due to decreasing oestrogen levels. If a couple enjoy an active sex life the woman is less likely to suffer vaginal symptoms. Some women may suffer loss of libido around the menopause. General health measures, and appropriate medical treatment will help to alleviate any distressing symptoms. Sexual desire need not be affected.

Hormone replacement therapy

When symptoms, due to lack of oestrogen, are severe, for example for frequent disabling hot flushes or for vaginitis, natural oestrogen with progestogen tablets are prescribed. The content of oestrogen in these pills is very much lower than the dose of synthetic oestrogen in the contraceptive pill. When hormone replacement therapy is being taken, there is less anxiety about the risks of heart disease and cancer.

A positive benefit of HRT is in the prevention of osteoporosis, a serious and frequently disabling condition. All women should discuss the indications for HRT with their doctors.

The majority of women will go through the menopause with very little difficulty, and will emerge somewhat enriched, more mature, and with a new sexual freedom. The absence of monthly periods and the knowledge that there is no possibility of pregnancy will be welcomed.

USE OF NATURAL FAMILY PLANNING DURING THE PRE-MENOPAUSE

The pre-menopause may last for as long as ten years for some women, from 45–55 years of age, for example. For other women it may only take two years from start to finish.

In addition to the physical and psychological problems of the pre-menopause (already discussed) there is the additional problem of family planning.

Many women fear the 'menopausal baby' with the well-documented increased risk of Down's Syndrome or Mongolism. In addition, there may be psychological problems created for the parents at a time in life when their offspring may be grown up and they feel unable to cope with an unplanned pregnancy. This fear may lead to reluctance to have sexual intercourse. As cycles become irregular, each month brings anxiety and this is increased when a period is missed. A pregnancy test may be done to give reassurance.

All women should realise that they become less fertile as they grow older. In countries where there is no family planning, the average time between the birth of the last child and the menopause is twelve years.

Dr Evelyn Billing quoted these figures:

In the age group 40–45 years, less than 35 per cent of women are still fertile. In the age group 45–50 years, less than 1 per cent of women are still fertile. Over 50 years pregnancy is rare. (These figures are given for women where no birth control method is used.)

If a woman has had previous experience in assessing her fertility prior to the pre-menopausal period, this is very valuable. It is possible to begin using natural family planning at this time, provided a woman is under close supervision from her NFP teacher.

The couple who have previously been prepared for periods of abstinence may find it easier to cope with the abstinence necessary in the pre-menopausal period. With good communication between a couple and a thorough knowledge of the changes taking place in a woman's body, this time can be made much easier.

The length of the pre-menopause and the severity of associated symptoms varies considerably between women. It may extend over months or years. Fertility may disappear then reappear months later. It is impossible to predict when fertility will end, although a woman's pattern may be similar to that of her mother or sisters.

It should be stressed that the menopause only marks the end of a woman's fertility; her femininity is unaffected.

CHANGES THAT CAN BE EXPECTED IN A WOMAN'S CYCLE

Variation in cycle length

Cycles may be shorter (ovulation occurs sooner) than usual – twenty-three days or less.

Ovulation could be delayed, resulting in a long cycle.

The post-ovulatory phase may be shortened (8–10 days), because of an inefficient corpus luteum and lower progesterone levels.

Anovulatory cycles

No temperature shift occurs in anovulatory cycles, which may vary in length.

There may be a pattern of dryness, or occasional patches of mucus.

Vaginal bleeding

There may be heavy prolonged menstrual flow with clots – the endometrium is overstimulated by the higher oestrogen levels which are caused by increased stimulation from the pituitary gland. Heavy bleeding may result in anaemia and fatigue.

Bleeding may be light and irregular. Though painful periods may have once been the rule, now many are painless.

Spotting may occur either between periods or in place of a true period.

Bleeding between periods sometimes coincides with ovulation. This is more common in long cycles.

True menstrual bleeding follows ovulation (shown by temperature shift) within 10–14 days. Any other bleeding may be associated with oestrogen activity, therefore that day could be fertile.

By recording her temperature daily, a woman will see why menstruation may be delayed, see what type of bleeding it is, and see if the cycle was ovulatory or not.

As a general rule:-

If periods are getting further apart, shorter and lighter – there is no reason to worry.

But if periods are getting closer together, longer and heavier, or if there is any bleeding between periods, medical advice must be sought. It may be due to hormone imbalance, but it should be investigated as there are many other causes.

RECORDING ON THE PRE-MENOPAUSAL CHART

1. Mucus signs are observed and recorded – dry days are infertile – marked in green with a 'D' on the chart. A basic infertile pattern of mucus should be marked in green with an 'M' added.

   A moist or sticky sensation occuring during otherwise dry days will denote the presence of mucus. These potentially fertile days are marked in yellow or with an 'M'. Any day on which fertile-type lubricative, transparent, stretchy mucus is noticed should be marked in yellow with an 'F'. Ovulation will be expected to follow the appearance of this peak mucus. Any day of bleeding, even blood spotting, should be marked in red or with a 'P'.
2. Changes in the cervix may be recorded.
3. The daily temperature is recorded.
4. Hot flushes and other symptoms of the pre-menopause – physical and emotional changes – should be noted.

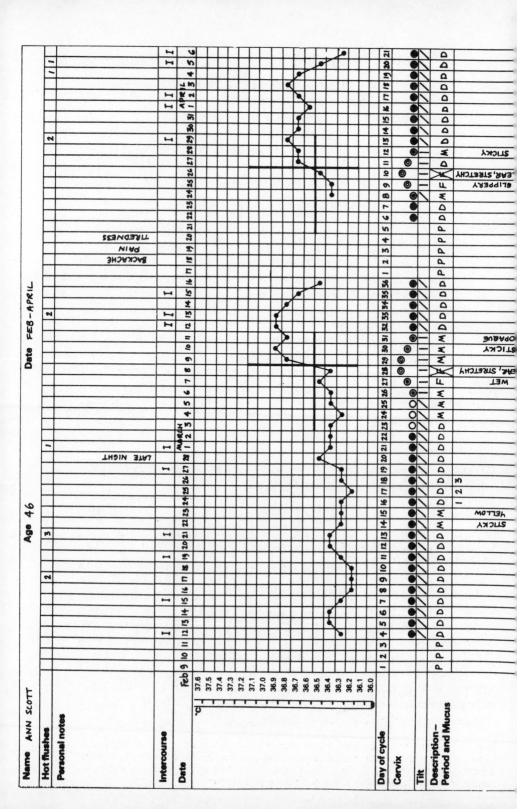

The special sixteen week pre-menopausal chart should be used to record as much information as possible about general health and progress through the change of life.

RECOGNISING SIGNS OF INFERTILITY

The recognition of infertility is as important as awareness of fertility in the pre-menopausal period.

1. Dry days. There may be long periods of dryness. There may be complete cycles with no mucus. Ovulation may occur, the temperature will show a biphasic pattern, but the cycle would be infertile because sperm would be unable to survive without mucus.
   Alternatively there may be a basic infertile pattern of sticky, crumbly mucus – a constant, unchanging pattern with no typical build-up to peak mucus.
2. The cervix will be low, firm, closed and tilted.
3. The temperature pattern will be monophasic (anovulatory).

RECOGNISING SIGNS OF FERTILITY

1. Appearance of any mucus or change in the basic infertile pattern of mucus may indicate the return of fertility. (Mucus becomes less and less as time goes on.)
2. The cervix will be high, soft, short, open and straight. As time goes by the cervix will cease to alter in this way.
3. The temperature pattern will be biphasic (ovulatory).

GUIDELINES FOR AVOIDING PREGNANCY DURING THE PRE-MENOPAUSE

Pre-ovulatory phase, and anovulatory cycles
Intercourse must be avoided on any day of blood loss.

Only dry days are considered infertile. A couple should abstain at the first sign of mucus.

A basic infertile pattern of mucus must be seen as a constant unchanging pattern for over two weeks, before being considered infertile. Any change from the basic infertile pattern of mucus may indicate returning fertility. A change is seen as an increasing amount or a change in any of the characteristics of the mucus.

Fig 13.1 Recording on the pre-menopausal chart. Part of a pre-menopausal chart to show the pattern of fertility and infertility shown by the temperature, mucus and cervical signs. Note that intercourse is restricted to the infertile phase according to the pre-menopausal guidelines. The number of hot flushes and other personal notes are also recorded

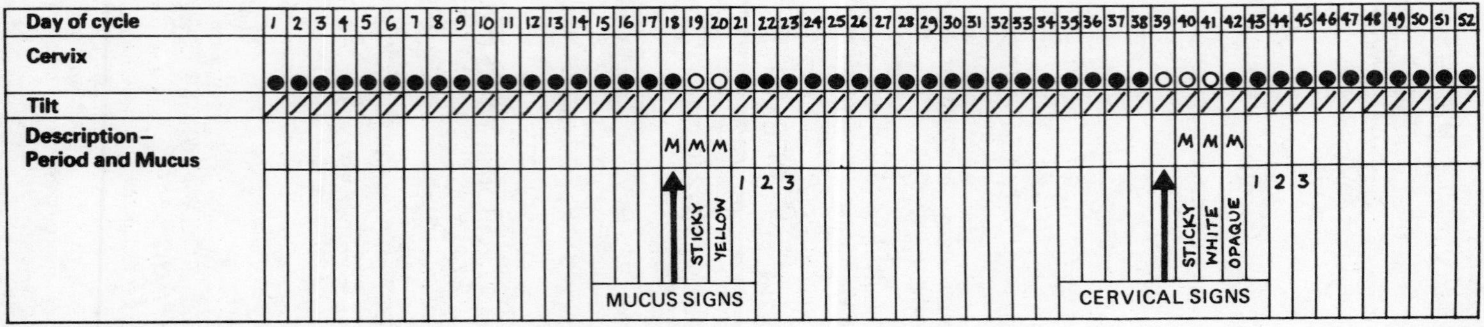

Day of cycle	1	2	3	4	5	6	7	8	9	10	11	12	13	14	15	16	17	18	19	20	21	22	23	24	25	26	27	28	29	30	31	32	33	34	35	36	37	38	39	40	41	42	43	44	45	46	47	48	49	50	51	52
Cervix	●	●	●	●	●	●	●	●	●	●	●	●	●	●	●	●	●	O	O	O	O	●	●	●	●	●	●	●	●	●	●	●	●	●	●	●	●	●	O	O	O	●	●	●	●	●	●	●	●	●	●	●
Tilt																																																				
Description – Period and Mucus																																																				

MUCUS SIGNS
STICKY YELLOW   W W W   1 2 3

CERVICAL SIGNS
STICKY WHITE   WHITE OPAQUE   W W W   1 2 3

Fig 13.2 Recording the earliest sign of fertility shown by the arrows indicating changes in the mucus or cervix

Anne Scott 46 January – July

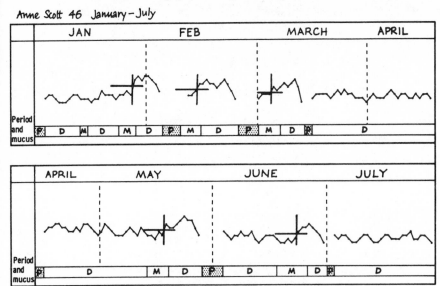

Fig 13.3 Two consecutive 16 week pre-menopausal charts recorded by a 46 year old woman. Note the irregular cycles, some showing evidence of ovulation and others are anovular

Anne Scott 51 May – December

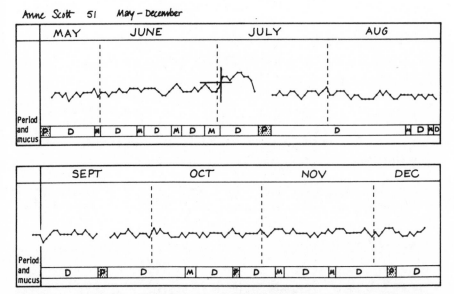

Fig 13.4 Post-menopausal infertility. 5 years later, there is only evidence of ovulation once, in July. Following this there are six months without further signs of ovulation. There were periods of blood loss, but little mucus. This woman will no longer be fertile, so charting may be discontinued.

Patches of mucus or blood spotting may occur during otherwise dry phases. These must be considered as potentially fertile.

Many pre-menopausal women find the earliest information about times of fertility and infertility is shown by the cervix. The earliest sign of change from the infertile pattern may indicate approaching fertility. This may be shown by either the cervix or the mucus. Intercourse must be avoided during the days the fertile signs last, and for three days after the infertile pattern has returned, as in figure 13.2.

It is wise to restrict intercourse to evenings only to allow any mucus to become apparent as the day progresses. Abstinence should be observed on the day following intercourse to prevent semen present in the vagina from masking mucus signs.

Post-ovulatory phase

Only the temperature chart will give definite information as to whether ovulation has occurred or not. Intercourse may be resumed following the third consecutive undisturbed high temperature past peak day.

Combined fertility is then zero, and intercourse day or night until the next menstruation carries no possibility of pregnancy.

EFFECTIVENESS DURING THE PRE-MENOPAUSE

If a couple choose to use the temperature rule alone, and limit intercourse to the post-ovulatory phase only, there is almost no chance of pregnancy, but there may be very long periods of abstinence.

If a woman is experienced in mucus and cervical signs, she may choose to use the pre-ovulatory phase for intercourse too. It should be understood that there is always a very slight chance of pregnancy in the pre-ovulatory phase.

There may be times when the pre-menopausal chart seems confusing. A couple should abstain throughout this time and continue charting patiently until a recognisable pattern of fertility or infertility emerges.

CONCLUSION

During a woman's life, there are three times of great physical and emotional change – at puberty, motherhood and the menopause. These times can be made easier if the changes are understood. Fertility awareness will encourage a positive approach to understanding and coping with these changes.

Gynaecology

14 Infertility and Subfertility

DEFINING FERTILITY PROBLEMS_____

An infertile couple is a couple who are unable to conceive after one year of regular intercourse. (Sterility is a term reserved for a couple who can never conceive.)

Subfertility denotes a reduced state of fertility, whereby some factors such as a low sperm count or damaged fallopian tubes may reduce the chances of conception.

It is now estimated that one in eight couples have fertility problems. The peak of fertility for both men and women occurs around 18–20 years. However, many couples are now choosing to use effective contraceptive methods to postpone their childbearing until later in life, for career or social reasons. The fact is that 75 per cent of women over thirty take two years or more to conceive their first child. Even when a couple of normal fertility have intercourse at the most fertile time in the cycle, it takes an average of three cycles for conception to occur.

In the light of the above figures, it will be apparent that many couples presenting with fertility problems will become pregnant without treatment in due course.

VALUE OF FERTILITY AWARENESS_____

A couple who use natural family planning and are familiar with the natural fertility cycle will be in a good position to detect any apparent changes in the fertility signs. Most couples who visit doctor's surgeries or infertility clinics will be asked to keep temperature charts, although the value of mucus signs is frequently either underestimated or not discussed at all.

Temperature charts are a valuable means of assessing whether ovulation is occurring. A biphasic chart is indicative of an ovulatory cycle, whereas a monophasic chart indicates the absence of ovulation and therefore an infertile cycle. Temperature charts also show the length of the post-ovulatory phase. If this is less than about nine days, then implantation will be disturbed and the cycle will be infertile.

Observation of cervical mucus provides the most accurate means of timing intercourse to optimise the chances of conception. Some women may have irregular cycles or fertile mucus signs may last only a matter of hours, in which case careful observation of cervical mucus and appropriate timing of intercourse is vital to achieve pregnancy.

DIANE AND TED: Diane and Ted had been trying for a baby for four years. They had been fully investigated at the fertility clinic, where there was said to be no apparent cause for infertility. Although a highly educated couple, they had very little understanding of their own physiology. At the first interview, it became apparent that Diane had irregular cycles (25–33 days). A hectic lifestyle including pressures at work resulted in infrequent intercourse. Increasing fertility awareness allowed Diane to experience the sensation of a very short mucus build-up, and time intercourse appropriately. She conceived in her second cycle of charting.

HOME KITS TO PREDICT OVULATION_____

The day before ovulation there is a sudden surge of luteinising hormone, LH (see page 31). This hormone can now be measured in simple home tests.

Clearplan One-Step is one such test in which a dipstick is held in a stream of urine first thing in the morning. A positive LH test shows a blue line after five minutes. First Response is a similar urine test, which identifies the LH surge by means of an easy-to-read colour change.

Tests are carried out for between five and ten days of the cycle, dependent on cycle length and regularity. They indicate the time of maximum fertility. As most women will ovulate within 12–24 hours of the positive test, intercourse during this time carries the highest chance of pregnancy. These kits do not define the limits of fertility, so cannot be used to avoid pregnancy.

Home kits are relatively expensive, but can be a valuable aid for women experiencing difficulty observing mucus symptom.

FACTORS INVOLVED IN CONCEPTION_____

If conception is to occur, the most important physiological conditions required are that a woman must ovulate, her fallopian tubes must be patent and her partner should have an adequate number of live normal sperm capable of penetrating the cervical mucus and subsequently meeting the ovum.

Any couple planning a pregnancy should be in good health. This is equally important for a couple with fertility problems.

THE CAUSE OF FERTILITY PROBLEMS

Infertility may be caused by problems in either partner or both. An estimated 40 per cent of infertility cases are found to be related to the woman, a further 40 per cent are found to originate in the man, 10 per cent of cases are caused by low fertility in both partners and in the remaining 10 per cent no cause will be found.

It is important that even when the major cause of infertility rests with one partner, the problem should be viewed as the problem of the couple rather than of an individual.

Many women delay childbearing until their late twenties or early thirties. A woman is at her most fertile between 20 and 28 years, when cycles tend to be regular and ovulatory. If fertility problems first present at 35, instead of 25, years, it is more difficult to treat because of the natural decline in fertility. The man's age is not a significant factor.

MALE INFERTILITY

The male partner may be infertile or subfertile as a result of various different factors. Fertility problems may be a consequence of infections such as sexually transmitted diseases, tuberculosis or orchitis (inflammation of the testes which may occur as a complication of mumps contracted after puberty). Certain drugs may reduce libido (sexual desire) and potency (virility) and may therefore affect fertility. These drugs include tranquillisers and some drugs used to treat high blood pressure. Drugs used in the treatment of cancer may impair sperm production.

the testes and impair sperm producton. This may also occur in men who wear very tight underpants or jeans, or men working in very high temperatures.

Some men may have congenital abnormalities of the reproductive tract or abnormalities in the male sex hormone or pituitary hormone systems.

General ill health, fatigue and stress may cause temporary infertility.

Psychological pressures may lead to sexual problems including impotence (failure to achieve or maintain an erection) and severe premature ejaculation. Psycho-sexual counselling may be warranted.

Finally some men may seek help to restore their fertility following surgical sterilisation (vasectomy). Although surgical reversal may appear successful, the presence of anti-sperm antibodies may prevent the return of fertility.

A thorough medical and physical examination will be carried out to exclude any apparent infections or abnormalities, and a specimen of seminal fluid will be analysed. If semen analyses show sperm of consistently poor quality or quantity, then further investigations will be required to determine the cause of the problem.

The treatment of male infertility is still in its infancy and at present is relatively ineffective. If the man if found to be infertile or subfertile, artificial insemination may be offered.

FEMALE INFERTILITY

Causes of infertility in women

Tubal damage
Tubal damage accounts for about one third of all cases of female infertility. The damage may be caused by infection, adhesions, tubal pregnancy, or as a result of sterilisation procedures.

a) Infection
The microscopic hairs lining the tubes are easily damaged by any pelvic infection. Salpingitis may occur following childbirth, abortion, sexually transmitted diseases (particularly gonorrhoea, chlamydia and non-specific urethritis), or following insertion of an intra-uterine contraceptive device. Tubal damage will impede the passage of the sperm and the ovum making conception unlikely.

b) Adhesions
These are bands of fibrous tissue in the pelvis that may develop after surgery, or following pelvic infection. They may prevent the release of the ovum or impede its passage to or within the tube.

c) Ectopic pregnancy
If conception occurs, the fertilised ovum may be unable to pass along the damaged tube which may have very poor muscular movement. The

embryo will continue to develop in the tube, resulting in a tubal or ectopic pregnancy. If this is undiagnosed, rupture of the tube may follow. A woman who has an ectopic pregnancy will complain of severe one-sided abdominal pain which may in some be accompanied by vaginal bleeding. This condition requires immediate surgical intervention.

d) Surgical sterilisation
Some women who have previously been sterilised may wish to regain their fertility (for example following remarriage or the death of a child). The extent of tubal damage incurred at the time of sterilisation will determine the chances of successful reversal.

Endometriosis
This is a condition where endometrial tissue grows in abnormal places such as on the surface of the ovaries, or within the fallopian tubes. It may prevent passage of the ovum from the ovary to the tube, or impede passage of the sperm or ovum within the tube. Endometriosis may be suspected if a woman develops pain at ovulation, before or during menstruation, or complains of discomfort during intercourse. A dark brown (chocolate) discharge is characteristic of endometriosis.

Hormonal imbalance
Imbalance of the female sex hormone or pituitary hormone systems may be responsible for the infertility. Excessive weight loss or anorexia nervosa may cause anovulation and secondary amenorrhoea.

Unruptured follical syndrome
Rarely a follicle may mature in the ovary but then for some reason fail to rupture. A corpus luteum will form and produce progesterone as indicated by the biphasic temperature chart. The length of the post-ovulatory phase will be variable – it may be of normal length, shortened or very long. This is known as the unruptured follicle syndrome.

Fibroids
These are abnormal growths of muscular tissue in the uterus which may block the tubes or impair implantation resulting in early miscarriage. Fibroids may cause heavy or painful periods.

Damaged cervix
Any operative treatment of the cervix may damage the mucus-producing crypts and lead to infertility.

An incompetent cervix is a term used to describe a cervix which is unable to provide sufficent support for pregnancy to continue beyond about 12–16 weeks and may therefore be a cause of recurrent miscarriages and subsequent childlessness.

Some drugs may impair production of cervical mucus. These include antihistamines used to dry up the secretions in a common cold or for hay fever or other allergic conditions, and anti-inflammatory drugs used in the treatment of rheumatism.

Chemical irritants such as vaginal deodorants alter the normal vaginal medium and provide a poor environment for sperm survival. The normal mucus pattern will be masked.

Miscarriage
Care should be taken in the early months of pregnancy to avoid strenuous or abnormal activity. It is wise to avoid intercourse at times when the period is due in the first three months. During pregnancy, unless a couple are medically advised otherwise, intercourse can take place as desired provided a woman feels comfortable. As the pregnancy advances couples may need to adapt their lovemaking positions to keep weight off the woman's abdomen.

Miscarriage or spontaneous abortion occurs most commonly around 10–14 weeks of pregnancy. There are many causes of miscarriage. There may be some abnormality of the foetus which arrests development. Incompetent cervix has been mentioned, but other abnormalities of the genital tract such as fibroids may be responsible. Hormone imbalance is a further cause, but most often the reason for the miscarriage is not diagnosed.

The miscarriage may be complete or incomplete. In the latter case a dilatation and curettage (D&C) will be performed to remove any retained products of conception. A pelvic examination is carried out about six weeks after a miscarriage, and normal physiology returns by 3 months. For many couples, miscarriage is a traumatic experience physically and psychologically. It is wise to wait for this time before planning a further pregnancy to allow time for recovery and readjustment.

KERRY AND IAN: Kerry, aged 30, had a two-year-old son, but had been trying to conceive for the past year. She complained of heavy delayed periods, which her consultant gynaecologist diagnosed as early miscarriages. This caused considerable distress. Following sympto-thermal charting, it became apparent that Kerry had very delayed ovulations. They had previously been timing intercourse around day 14, the day they thought was the most fertile time. By learning to recognise her mucus symptom, Kerry realised that her fertile phase was much later and conceived following intercourse on day 23, the day before peak day.

Physical or emotional stress may affect fertility

The effect of stress on the menstrual cycle has already been discussed. A common reaction to stress is to delay ovulation. The mucus build-up will be interrupted and the temperature shift will likewise be delayed, resulting in a long cycle. Severe stress may completely suppress ovulation, resulting in anovulatory cycles and subsequent infertility. Increasing anxiety and the stress of infertility investigations may exacerbate the problem.

Some women may so desperately want a child that they have a phantom pregnancy. This is a situation where a woman believes she is pregnant and has signs and symptoms of early pregnancy. Menstruation will stop and she may begin to produce breast milk. A woman in this state has a temporarily imbalanced hormone state and would be unable to conceive before her hormone balance had been restored.

Occasionally a couple may appear infertile, but when investigated further, the woman may express ambivalent feelings about having a baby. She may be avoiding intercourse at the fertile time. Specialised counselling is warranted to help a couple who obviously have personal and relationship problems rather than clinical infertility. Psychological problems are rarely a primary cause of infertility, but more commonly arise from the stress of infertility.

Idiopathic infertility

This is a term used to describe a situation in which there is no apparent cause of infertility. After thorough investigation, about 10 per cent of infertile couples will be told that with the present state of knowledge there is no specific reason to explain their infertility.

Investigation of female infertility

Medical history and examination

A couple will usually be seen together initially, then both partners may be seen individually, when personal questions can be asked to establish previous sexual history, including any past history of sexually transmitted disease of which the partner may be unaware. A woman will be asked about previous pregnancies including abortions, and a man may be asked about any previous children he believes he has fathered. These details, which form a vital part of the infertility investigations, are treated with the strictest confidence throughout.

A thorough medical and gynaecological examination will be done to exclude obvious abnormalities and infections. This will frequently include a vaginal examination and cervical smear.

Blood tests

Blood tests may be done to measure female and male sex hormones and pituitary hormone levels. Oestrogen and progesterone levels are measured. The progesterone levels are estimated in the second half of the cycle, to give an indication as to whether ovulation has occurred and whether the corpus luteum is producing sufficient progesterone to sustain pregnancy. Follicle-stimulating hormone and luteinising hormone levels may be measured and the prolactin level may be checked. An excess of prolactin will block ovulation (compare the effect during breast-feeding). Several measurements of prolactin may be made because anxiety may affect the levels. The blood may also be tested for rubella (German measles) antibodies at this stage.

Temperature (and mucus) charts

Initial investigations of female infertility will include charting fertility symptoms. A thorough knowledge of fertility awareness is a great asset to a couple if they can be taught at this stage. Unfortunately, though a temperature chart is used to show the occurrence of ovulation, all too often the significance of cervical mucus is not discussed with the client.

Cervical mucus tests

A specimen of cervical mucus is taken at the appropriate time to estimate its fertile characteristics. The amount, the appearance and the texture of the mucus, including the Spinnbarkeit test and the ferning effect produced by fertile mucus are checked.

The post-coital test in the pre-ovulatory phase provides important information on the compatibility between the sperm and cervical mucus.

Hysterosalpingogram

This is a special X-ray technique used to assess the state of the fallopian tubes. A radio-opaque dye is passed through the cervix into the uterus and fallopian tubes. If the tubes are blocked, the dye will not pass into the abdomen. Sometimes the action of passing the dye may be sufficient to clear the tubes.

Laparoscopy

This is a technique used to view the ovaries, tubes and uterus, by an instrument known as a laparoscope. Laparoscopy is usually performed under general anaesthesia and involves two incisions, one just below the umbilicus and the other on the pubic hair line. This allows the organs to be manipulated into view. While the fallopian tubes are in view, a dye may be passed through the cervix to check for blockages in the tubes. If the tubes are patent, the dye will be seen to pass into the abdominal cavity.

Laparoscopy is generally performed in preference to a hysterosalpingogram, after 12-18 months of infertility. Fibroids, adhesions, endometriosis and tubal damage may all be diagnosed by laparoscopy.

Ultrasound scanning

Pelvic ultrasound scanning can be used as an aid to diagnosing the cause of infertility. A scan will reveal the size and position of the uterus, tubes and ovaries. It will also show the thickness of the endometrium and any uterine fibroids or ovarian cysts. The scan may be used to monitor the growth and maturation of ovarian follicles and to observe ovulation. If conception occurs, a scan will assist in the diagnosis of early pregnancy and can be used to monitor the development of the unborn child.

Treatment of female infertility

Treatment may be by surgical intervention or hormonal therapy. If ovulation is not occurring, fertility drugs such as clomiphene (Clomid) are frequently successful in inducing ovulation and subsequent pregnancy, but the side effects must be borne in mind. Overstimulation of the ovaries may lead to abdominal pain and cysts on the ovaries, requiring that the treatment be discontinued. The phenomenon of multiple births following the use of fertility drugs is widely known, although this is less common with the newer drugs and careful monitoring of the dosage.

The test-tube baby technique (*in vitro* fertilisation or IVF) is used as a means of bypassing blocked or damaged tubes.

The technique of *in vitro* (in glass) fertilisation and embryo transfer involves a lot of stress for the couple as the treatment programme is extensive. The treatment basically involves careful monitoring of the cycle to determine the time of ovulation (using all available means including ultrasound). Fertility drugs are used to ensure that several ova will reach maturity at which time they can be retrieved via laparoscopy or via a special needle through the abdominal wall guided by the use of ultrasound.

A fresh sample of the husband's sperm is then placed with the ova and observed. If fertilisation is successful, the embryos are grown to the 2–4 cell stage which takes about three days, at which time they will be transferred via a catheter through the cervix high up into the uterus.

The stimulation of several ova to maturity is necessary in an attempt to achieve at least three embryos – the optimum number required to achieve successful implantation and the maximum chance of pregnancy. (It is rare for all three embryos to implant successfully.)

There are obvious ethical issues involved with these techniques. Only about one in four embryos transfer successfully and there is the constant dilemma of wastage of embryos grown in the laboratory.

EMOTIONAL EFFECTS OF INFERTILITY ON A COUPLE

Couples who are faced with infertility may go through a series of emotional changes. The reactions may follow a similar pattern to that following bereavement. There may be grief for the loss of fertility just as one may grieve a lost relative or friend.

The first reaction may be one of surprise when the pregnancy does not follow as planned after birth control measures are stopped. The couple may deny both to themselves and others that they are trying for a baby and consequently delay in seeking help. They may become socially isolated if their friends are raising young families. If one partner longs for a child more than the other, this can create tension and further isolaton within the relationship.

Unexpected feelings of anger may be directed towards friends with young families and the medical personnel involved in the couple's infertility investigations and treatment. The long wait for appointments, test results, and treatment creates more frustration and anger.

If their general practitioner is aware of such problems, he/she can give support throughout this time by being available for discussions and explanations of the procedures being undertaken.

There may be feelings aroused by the loss of control over their lives as their privacy is invaded and sex loses its spontaneity. At the start of each period a woman may be flooded by feelings of depression, a sense of failure yet again and possibly anger towards her husband if he does not sympathise.

Fertility problems inevitably create anxiety, but it should be realised that tension can in turn contribute to failure to conceive.

Couples should know that they share a common experience with many others. One couple in eight experiences fertility problems, but the number remaining childless is small. Sadly there will be couples who have to adjust to a life without children. Adoption is an option for some, whereas others may choose to live a child-free life, frequently not losing all hope, as there are constantly new developments in this field.

15 Contraception, Sterilisation and Abortion

This section on contraception is intended to give an outline of other available methods of birth control. There is a constant stream of information available to the contraceptive user, through all areas of the media, some of which is useful and some of which is misleading, inaccurate, or frightening. The aim of this section is to give some of the facts about artificial contraception.

The relative effectiveness of contraceptive methods is shown in the table below. Each method will then be discussed in more detail including use of the method, effectiveness and associated side effects.

Fig 15.1 Relative effectiveness of contraceptive methods

Contraceptive method	Relative effectiveness
Sterilisation	
Combined pill	Highly effective
Sympto-thermal (post-ovulatory only)	
Intra-uterine device	
Progestogen only pill	
Condom	Effective
Diaphragm/cap	
Sympto-thermal (both phases)	
Spermicides alone	Not very effective
Withdrawal	Depends very much on the users
Douching	Ineffective

THE ORAL CONTRACEPTIVE PILL

The contraceptive pill remains the most popular method of reversible contraception. It is possibly also the most controversial method, frequently receiving widespread adverse publicity. There are basically three types of oral contraceptive pill:

1. The combined pill which contains two steroids, synthetic oestrogen and progestogen, is taken as a constant dose for 21 days out of 28.

   Phasic pills have been introduced with the objective of reducing the amount of hormone at certain times in the cycle, thus reducing the adverse side effects while maintaining the efficacy of the combined pill.

2. The biphasic and triphasic combined pills are two- and three-phase combined pills combining varying doses of oestrogen and a step-wise increase in progestogen to mimic the normal pattern of hormone secretion. They are taken 21 days out of 28.

3. The progestogen-only pill or mini-pill is taken every day without a break. It has fewer associated side effects, but shows a higher failure rate than the combined pills.

All types of oral-contraceptive pill interfere with the normal physiology of a woman's body.

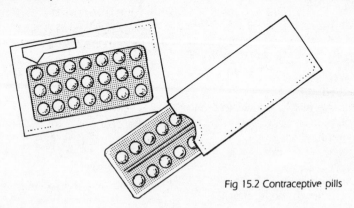

Fig 15.2 Contraceptive pills

The combined pill – oestrogen and progestogen (as 1 and 2 above)

Action
The main action of the combined pill is to suppress the normal control of the menstrual cycle or sex hormone system thus blocking the process leading to ovulation. It does this in two ways.

1. FSH is reduced, and thus the follicles are prevented from ripening and the ovum from maturing.
2. The LH surge is stopped, so the ovum is not released.

Other back-up effects of the combined pill make pregnancy unlikely even if an ovum is released. (This occurs most commonly when pills are forgotten.)

3. The progestogen component of the combined pill prevents sperm from entering the uterus by stimulating the production of thick barrier-type mucus.
4. It prevents implantation of the fertilised ovum by altering the state of the endometrium.
5. There may be some effect on the fallopian tubes, making them function less well in the transport of the ovum towards the uterus.

As a woman's normal cycle is suppressed, normal menstrual periods will be replaced by a hormone withdrawal bleed after the pills are stopped. While the pills are taken, the synthetic hormones build up the endometrium, although its structure differs and it is thinner than during a normal cycle. After the pill is stopped, the thin endometrium is shed, usually resulting in less bleeding which is often darker than a normal period. Withdrawal bleeds are usually less painful than normal menstrual periods.

Effectiveness
Combined pills are the most effective forms of contraception. The method failure rate is around 0.05 per cent. The user failure rate, usually as a result of forgotten pills, is less than 1 per cent.

Advantages
Provided the pills are taken as directed, it is an extremely effective method.
It may relieve anxiety about unplanned pregnancy.
It allows spontaneous intercourse throughout the cycle.
There is no direct relationship between intercourse and the contraceptive method.
Periods are usually shorter, lighter and less painful.
Symptoms of pre-menstrual syndrome may be relieved.

Disadvantages
If a combined pill is taken more than twelve hours late, the contraceptive effectiveness is reduced.
Breakthrough bleeding may occur if pills are missed.
Vomiting or diarrhoea may affect the absorption of the pill.

Other drugs, including some painkillers, antibiotics, sedatives and drugs to treat epilepsy and arthritis may affect the efficacy of the pill. Any woman prescribed medication should ensure that her doctor knows that she is taking the contraceptive pill.

It is suspected that the pill may alter the effect of other drugs such as those used in the treatment of diabetes and depression.

The normally acid medium of the vagina is altered in such a way that vaginal infections, such as thrush, are more common.

Medical supervision is required. A woman should have regular six-monthly check-ups of blood pressure and weight.

The return of fertility may be delayed following discontinuance of the pill. Some of the long term consequences of taking the pill may still be unknown.

Hormonal contraceptives have many well documented side effects. Widespread publicity of these effects may cause anxiety in some women. In some circumstances it may be difficult to differentiate between the hormonal effects and those induced by fear and anxiety.

Minor side effects attributed to the pill
Side effects commonly occur particularly during the first few cycles of pill-taking as the body adjusts to the increased level of hormones. Some of these effects are similar to those experienced in the early weeks of pregnancy and may disappear after the first two or three cycles. Although the side effects are frequently considered of nuisance value only, nevertheless if they are a cause of concern to a woman she should seek advice.

Women taking the pill may experience nausea and vomiting, fluid retention or increased appetite leading to weight gain. Some women may complain of headaches particularly during the pill-free week. Other side effects include breast discomfort, inter-menstrual spotting, tiredness, irritability, depression and loss of libido. Some women who wear contact lenses may suffer irritation from their lenses.

Major complications associated with pill use
i. Cardiovascular disease
The oestrogen component of the combined pill has been linked to an increase in the incidence of cardiovascular disease. Other factors including age (over 35 years) heavy smoking and obesity further increase the risk.

Blood clots or thromboses may develop in any veins or arteries, the severity of the problem depending on the location of the clot. The most commonly affected veins are the deep veins in the legs causing venous thrombosis.

Very rarely, a blood clot may form in the arteries supplying the heart or the brain, resulting in a coronary thrombosis or a cerebral haemorrhage, which could lead to permanent disability or death.

Women taking the pill should be alert to any possible warning signs of serious complications. These include the following cardiovascular signs:

Severe pain in the calf of one leg, especially if accompanied by swelling.
Severe central chest pain, or severe sharp pains in the chest, usually one-sided and aggravated by breathing.
Unexplained breathlessness, or cough with blood-stained phlegm.
Severe abdominal pain.
Any unusually frequent or severe prolonged headaches.
Fainting attacks or loss of consciousness.
Numbness or sudden weakness or very marked tingling affecting one side or one part of the body, (eg one arm or one side of the face or tongue).
Sudden visual or speech disturbance.

ii. Liver tumours
The incidence of tumours of the liver is increased in long-term pill users. Signs which may indicate liver disease include a severe generalised rash, which may be painful and jaundice or yellowing of the skin or eyes.

iii. Cancer of the cervix and breast
There is some anxiety about the increased risk of cancer of the cervix and breast. Among women who have taken the pill for more than five years, there is an increase in the number of abnormal cervical smears and cancer of the cervix. This may also be related to a sexually transmitted virus.

There are conflicting reports on the relation of the pill to breast cancer, but progestogen-only pill users are thought to be at higher risk. All women taking contraceptive pills should have regular cervical smears and breast examinations.

There is some evidence to suggest that the pill protects women from cancer of the ovaries and the endometrium.

The progestogen-only pill (mini-pill)

Action

The effect of the progestogen-only pill is mainly on the cervical mucus. It produces a thick barrier-type mucus which prevents passage of sperm into the uterus. Ovulation occurs in around 50 per cent of cycles. If the barrier effect fails and conception occurs, there is a further back-up effect, because the state of the endometrium is altered to prevent implantation.

Effectiveness

The progestogen-only pill, because of its mode of action, is slightly less effective than the combined pill. It has a user failure rate of around 1–4 per cent. The efficacy depends largely on the pill being taken regularly every single day of the cycle and at the same time of day regardless of bleeding. Although a couple can assume continuous protection if the pill is taken regularly, the maximum effectiveness is achieved if the pill is taken several hours before the usual time of intercourse. The effect on the mucus is at its maximum about 4–5 hours after it is taken.

The lower failure rate of 1 per cent applies to women over thirty-five years old, whose natural fertility is reduced. The progestogen-only pill is therefore a highly effective method for women in this category. Younger, highly fertile women would be assured of greater effectivenss with the combined pill.

Advantages

Provided the pills are taken as directed it is effective against pregnancy.
It allows spontaneous intercourse throughout the cycle.
There is no direct relationship between intercourse and the contraceptive method.
It is probably medically safer than the combined pill, as there is no oestrogenic effect and reduced progestogen.
It is often recommended during breastfeeding, although some authorities are concerned about the effect of the hormone on breast milk.
It can be used by women in the older age group and others where the combined pill is not recommended or is proving unsatisfactory.

Disadvantages

Irregular bleeding is the main problem associated with the progestogen-only pill. The periods may be more frequent, longer or shorter. Inter-menstrual bleeding may occur. In some women there will be no bleeding. Pills should be continued throughout as directed. If six weeks elapse with no period, especially if pills have been missed, a woman should see her doctor who will arrange a pregnancy test. If pregnancy is confirmed, pills should be discontinued immediately. There is no reliable evidence to link pill use during pregnancy with an increased incidence of congenital defects, but it is a wise precaution to avoid all drugs.

The pill *must* be taken regularly. If it is taken more than three hours late, the contraceptive effectiveness is reduced.

If a woman vomits within two hours of pill taking and is unable to keep another pill down within three hours, this must be considered as a missed pill. Similarly, diarrhoea may affect the absorption of the pill. The efficacy is probably reduced by the same drugs that affect the combined pill, for example some antibiotics and sedatives.

Fertility usually returns promptly after discontinuance of the progestogen-only pill, especially if a woman has been having periods fairly regularly, as these are an indication of ovulation and fertility. If periods do not return within six months, medical advice should be sought.

Because the progestogen-only pill does not invariably prevent conception, but has an action in preventing implantation, there may be moral or religious objections to its use.

Side effects associated with the progestogen-only pill
Little is known about side effects, especially long term, although most of the evidence is reassuring. Compared with the side effects of the combined pill they are much less common. Some women may complain of such symptoms as weight gain, loss of libido, breast tenderness, headache and dizziness. There is no associated increase in cardiovascular disease and the body systems including liver and thyroid, and blood levels of vitamins, minerals, sugar and fat seem to be less affected than by even the lowest dose of the combined pill.

Major complications
The incidence of tubal or ectopic pregnancy is increased, but this is still very rare. In women taking the progestogen-only pill, ovulation and conception may still occur. The slowing-down effect of progestogen on the fallopian tubes increases the chance of the fertilised ovum getting held up in the tube. This results in severe pain in the lower abdomen, usually one-sided. Any woman who suffers abdominal pain after a delayed, light or missed period should consult her doctor immediately. There is serious concern that women who have taken the progestogen-

only pill for more than five years are at a higher risk of developing breast cancer.

INJECTABLE HORMONAL CONTRACEPTIVES – DEPO-PROVERA

Depo-Provera is a long-acting progestogen (a synthetic progesterone-like substance) that is injected into a muscle. Its contraceptive effect lasts for three months. Its use is generally restricted to women who have just been immunised against rubella, in whom pregnancy within three months could have catastrophic effects on the foetus. It is also used in circumstances where a woman's partner has undergone vasectomy, to provide contraceptive cover until the seminal fluid is free from sperm.

Its appropriateness for women in lower social groups and for mentally handicapped women is a controversial issue, because of its possible administration without consent or adequate counselling about the potential risks.

The main side effect of Depo-Provera is menstrual chaos, particularly after the first injection. Periods may be heavy, irregular, or absent. Long-term use of Depo-Provera frequently causes amenorrhoea (absence of menstruation), which some women may find beneficial.

A newer injectable progestogen is Noristerat. It appears to cause less problem with bleeding, but must be given every eight weeks to provide contraceptive cover.

Other side effects similar to those with progestogen-only pills may occur, particularly weight gain.

Once administered the effect will last for at least three months and there is no way of reversing the action, even if side effects occur. There may be a delay in the return of fertility.

Injectable contraceptives provide protection against pregnancy comparable to the combined oral contraceptive pill.

THE INTRA-UTERINE CONTRACEPTIVE DEVICE (IUCD)

The intra-uterine contraceptive device, or coil, is a plastic, or plastic and metal device which is inserted through the cervix into the uterus by a doctor. All devices have a fine filament or thread attached, which protrudes from the cervix into the top of the vagina where it can be checked.

Action
The action of the coil is not completely understood. It was thought to act by altering the state of the endometrium in such a way that implantation was unlikely to take place. However, recent research has questioned this and has suggested that it may act earlier by preventing fertilisation.

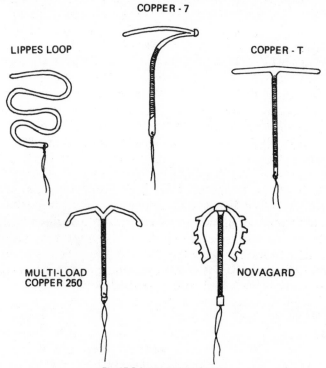

Fig 15.3 Intra-uterine devices

Plastic devices, for example the Lippes loop are relatively large and tend to increase the average menstrual loss. They may be left in place indefinitely for ten years or longer.

Coils wound with fine copper wire, release copper ions which probably inhibit enzymes vital to implantation. These devices are smaller and have a lower incidence of excessive bleeding. Copper-containing devices such as the Copper-7, Copper-T and Multi-load Copper 250 must be changed every 2–3 years according to the manufacturer's instructions as their efficiency is reduced after this time.

Novagard or Nova T is a copper-containing device with a silver core, which can be left in place for up to five years. The choice of device is made by the doctor taking into account the woman's personal and gynae-cological history and future contraceptive needs. Every woman should know which device she has been fitted with and when it should be replaced.

Effectiveness
Effectiveness during the first year varies from 1–7 per cent on the Pearl Index.

The variation in effectiveness is attributed to the various types of device, the ease of insertion, expulsion (especially during the first period after insertion), and a woman's ability to detect expulsion of the device. The expulsion rate is higher for women who have not had children.

Advantages
A woman should be unaware of the presence of her coil. Apart from checking the threads, no further action need be taken during the time it is in place, and therefore it allows spontaneous intercourse at any time in the cycle.

IRENE AND JACK: Irene is one of the few unhappy women who found her life in ruins after having her family curtailed prematurely. She and Jack had one son but longed for a daughter. They decided to wait for a while after the birth of their son before planning another pregnancy. She developed complications on the pill and so was advised to have a coil fitted, but then suffered severe haemorrhages and later needed a hysterectomy. 'I am angry because no one explained anything to me, and I didn't know there could be complications like this. I can't bear to think how ignorant I was about my body.' Irene believes that fertility awareness should be part of every girl's education.

Disadvantages

The device is usually inserted during a period. There may be some pain on insertion and for a few hours afterwards. Abdominal cramps and backache may be caused by attempts of the uterine muscles to expel the device.

Heavy, prolonged, painful periods may result.

Some women may experience spotting between periods.

The device may be expelled. This may be accompanied by pain or bleeding, but can happen without a woman's knowledge. After every period a woman should check the threads of her coil, at the cervix, to ensure that it is still in position.

There is an increased risk of pelvic infection in all coil users. Any abnormal pain or tenderness in the abdomen, pain during or after intercourse, or an offensive discharge, should be reported to a doctor, especially if accompanied by a fever. Infection may spread, causing damage to the fallopian tubes, resulting in infertility. Women who have had at least one child are generally more suited to the method than younger nulliparous women, whose future fertility may be at stake.

Perforation of the uterus. This is a very rare but dangerous complication usually occurring at the time of insertion.

If the IUCD fails and pregnancy results, a woman will need special attention because

a) Conception with a coil in place increases the risk of ectopic (tubal) pregnancy. This may lead to rupture of the tube after several weeks and surgical removal.

b) Any woman who has a missed period accompanied by abdominal pain should see her doctor.

c) If a woman becomes pregnant with a coil in place, there is a higher risk of miscarriage either if it is left in place, or at the time of removal though, in either case, the pregnancy can proceed normally

If pregnancy is desired, the coil must be removed by a doctor, after which fertility will usually return quickly. A woman can be taught to recognise her fertility symptoms while her coil is still in place.

There may be moral or religious objections to the use of an IUCD because of the possibility of an egg being fertilised, but unable to develop further, ie it may have an abortifacient effect.

IUCD's are contra-indicated for women who have never been pregnant or have a history of sexually transmitted disease.

BARRIER METHODS

Use of barrier methods is increasing because they provide some protection against sexually transmitted diseases including HIV (AIDS).

The diaphragm

The diaphragm or Dutch cap is a soft rubber dome-shaped device with a flexible metal spring reinforcing the rim.

Action

The diaphragm is inserted into the vagina in such a way that the cervix is completely covered. It is held in place by the spring tension of the rim and the vaginal muscles. The front of the diaphragm rests on the pubic bone. When properly positioned the diaphragm will prevent access of the sperm to the cervix. It does not fit tightly enough to prevent access to all sperm, so a spermicidal cream or jelly must be used with it.

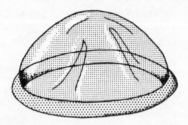

Fig 15.4 The diaphragm

Effectiveness

The method effectiveness is 3 per cent. The use effectiveness is 6–20 per cent. The wide variation in user failure rate may be an indication that some couples find the device in some way unacceptable, and therefore it is not used consistently.

Advantages

When properly used it is highly effective.

It need not interfere with lovemaking as the diaphragm and spermicide may be inserted up to three hours before intercourse.

When the diaphragm is properly positioned, it should not be felt by the user or her partner. It should stay in place and be comfortable during all everyday activities.

It is medically safe – there is no physiological disturbance to the menstrual cycle.

It is used only when needed.

Its use during menstruation may make intercourse more acceptable.
The spermicides give extra lubrication during intercourse.
It can be used during breastfeeding.

Disadvantages

A woman needs to be well motivated to use it.
It must be fitted initially by a trained person who will give thorough instruction in the use of the method.
It needs checking every 6–12 months, following childbirth or miscarriage, and if a woman gains or loses more than 7lb in weight.
Spermicides are ineffective after three hours. Additional spermicide should be used (usually in the form of a pessary) if there is an interval of more than three hours between the time the device is inserted and the time of intercourse.
The diaphragm must stay in place for at least six hours, but not more than twenty-four hours before it is removed, washed and dried carefully.
It should be inspected regularly by holding it up to the light and checking for faults.
Some men claim it can be felt during intercourse.
It may be viewed by some women with distaste.
The spontaneity of lovemaking may be marred unless a couple are relaxed and comfortable about the use of the device.
Side effects of the diaphragm and spermicides include irritation of the vagina, allergy to the rubber and vaginal infections.
Some women are unable to use this method because of anatomical variations which may only become apparent when the device is first fitted by a professional.

Cervical cap

A cervical cap may be used in preference to the larger diaphragm. A cap fits snugly over the cervix, held on by suction. Spermicides should be used in conjunction with this. A cervical cap may be preferred if a male partner complains that a diaphragm can be felt during intercourse. A cap must be properly fitted by a trained person, when instruction will be given on use of the method.

The contraceptive or 'Today' sponge

'Today' is a round, soft polythene sponge with a depression on one side that fits over the cervix and a loop for ease of removal. It is impregnated with spermicide which kills sperm on contact for up to 48 hours regardless of the number of acts of intercourse. After this time, and not less than six hours after the last intercourse, the sponge is removed and thrown away.

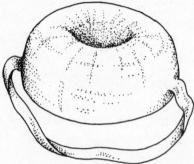

Fig 15.5 The contraceptive sponge

The sponge, which has proved very popular with women in America, is available from chemists or free of charge from family planning clinics in the UK. The one-size disposable sponge acts rather like a tampon in that it adapts to fit each user. The failure rate is higher than an individually fitted diaphragm. Recent trials by Family Health International in many countries including America and the UK reported use effectiveness ranging from 9–27 per cent.

The sheath or condom

The condom is a thin rubber sheath that is worn over the erect penis during sexual intercourse. It must be put on before there is any contact between the penis and the vulva. A condom prevents semen from being deposited in the vagina. Many condoms are impregnated with spermicidal lubricants to increase the effectiveness.

Use of the sheath

The teat end (or closed end) of the sheath should be held between the thumb and forefinger to expel the air. The sheath is then carefully unrolled over the full length of the erect penis, ensuring that the last half inch of the teat end is left empty at the tip of the penis to collect the semen. The sheath must be held in place on the erect penis when withdrawing from the vagina after ejaculation.

Effectiveness

Method effectiveness – 3 per cent; use effectiveness – 5–15 per cent.

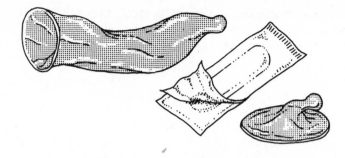

Fig 15.6 The sheath

Rupture of reputable brands of condoms is a very rare occurrence. The variable use-effectiveness figures generally denote poor technique and inconsistent use of the sheath.

Advantages
It allows a man to assume birth control responsibility.
Sheaths are reliable when used properly with a spermicide, at every act of intercourse.
They are easily obtainable from chemists and other stores.
Sheaths give some protection against sexually transmitted diseases.
A sheath may help to control premature ejaculation.

Disadvantages
Foreplay is interrupted to put on the sheath. Some couples may prefer the woman to put the sheath on her partner's penis as part of the lovemaking.
The man must withdraw rapidly following ejaculation, before his erection is lost.
The sheath may reduce sensitivity of the glans penis.
There may be an allergy to the rubber or the spermicide. (Anti-allergic sheaths are now available.)
Sheaths can only be used for one act of intercourse and should not be used after the expiry date marked on the packet.

Spermicides
Spermicides are chemical substances which act by immobilising sperms, leaving them unlikely to be able to cause fertilisation. They are placed high in the vagina in the form of pessaries, foams, gels or creams.

The newer contraceptive film or C-film is a semi-transparent square of soluble spermicidal film. It is packed between squares of silver foil for ease of handling. Contraceptive film has the advantage of being less messy to use.

Spermicides used alone are unreliable in preventing pregnancy. They should only be used in conjunction with a sheath or diaphragm as advised by a doctor.

Spermicide may cause minor irritations or allergies in either partner.

Only recommended spermicides should be used, because some spermicides, as well as oil-based lubricants and certain medicated pessaries, such as Canesten, will damage the rubber of diaphragms and condoms.

Spermicides containing Nonoxynol have been shown to inactivate HIV (AIDS virus).

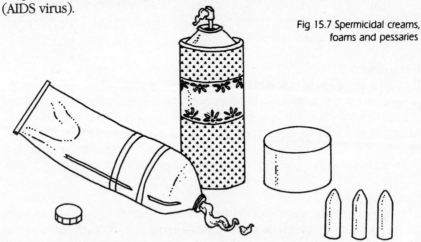

Fig 15.7 Spermicidal creams, foams and pessaries

Barrier methods and natural family planning

Is it possible to combine barrier methods with natural methods? This question is always asked. In fact it is true that those using barrier methods certainly do not need to do so on every day in the cycle.

In some clinics the recommendation is made that barriers should be used after menstruation, through the pre-ovulatory period, until the third high temperature is recorded on the chart. However, the use of diaphragms and spermicidal cream or foam make the recognition of the mucus symptom difficult if not impossible.

It is interesting that many experienced users of natural methods say that they prefer not to rely on the barrier methods of contraception on days of maximum fertility.

COITUS INTERRUPTUS OR WITHDRAWAL

Coitus interruptus is not a reliable method of birth control. If a man is to use the withdrawal method effectively he must withdraw his penis from his partner's vagina before he reaches orgasm and ejaculate well away from her vulva. However, sperm may be released before ejaculation in the pre-ejaculatory fluid and this may result in pregnancy. Withdrawal is generally found to be an unsatisfactory method for both partners, and can cause considerable anxiety.

EMERGENCY CONTRACEPTION

Post-coital contraception is an emergency measure used, for example, in cases of sheath failure, or unprotected intercourse. Depending on the position in the cycle, it acts by preventing fertilisation or implantation.

Hormone pills as a post-coital method

If it is established that there is a risk of unplanned pregnancy, the doctor may prescribe two high dose combined pills to be taken immediately and a further two pills to be taken twelve hours later. The first dose must be taken within seventy-two hours of a single act of unprotected intercourse.

Many women will feel very sick after taking these pills because of the high oestrogen content. Further advice should be sought if vomiting occurs as the tablets will need repeating.

The intra-uterine device as a post-coital method

In some circumstances, a woman may be fitted with an intra-uterine device or coil. The device must be fitted within five days of exposure to pregnancy to prevent implantation of the fertilised ovum. This method is contra-indicated for young women who have not borne children or where there may have been exposure to sexually transmitted disease, for example in cases of rape. This is because of the increased risk of pelvic inflammatory disease in coil users. It may be a suitable method for older women of proven fertility, especially if the coil is chosen for long-term contraceptive use.

The overall failure rate for post-coital pills is around 1 per cent, but no pregnancies have been recorded using the intra-uterine device as a post-coital method.

UNPLANNED PREGNANCIES

Although contraception is widely available in this country, unplanned pregnancies do occur either as a result of contraceptive failure, or from unprotected intercourse. Unplanned pregnancies are not necessarily unwanted, and may in fact result in much-loved and wanted children.

There are three options open for a couple faced with an unplanned pregnancy:

1. To continue with the pregnancy and keep the baby.
2. To continue with the pregnancy and have the baby adopted. This option may be preferred by some young girls in a situation where they are unable to care for the child.
3. Termination of pregnancy or abortion.

ABORTION

Laws relating to abortion vary enormously in different countries. In England, abortion is legal for the following reasons:

1. The continuance of the pregnancy would involve risk to the life of the pregnant woman greater than if the pregnancy were terminated;
2. The continuance of the pregnancy would involve risk of injury to the physical or mental health of the pregnant woman greater than if the pregnancy were terminated;
3. The continuance of the pregnancy would involve risk of injury to the physical or mental health of the existing child(ren) of the family of the pregnant woman greater than if the pregnancy were terminated;
4. There is substantial risk that if the child were born it would suffer from such physical or mental abnormalities as to be seriously handicapped.

Thorough counselling is essential before an abortion is performed, to explore the woman's/couple's feelings about the pregnancy, and the effects fo the abortion in both the short and long term.

Before seven weeks of pregnancy, that is seven weeks after the first day of the last menstrual period, some authorities may use prostaglandin gel vaginally, and oral tablets, on an outpatient basis. There will be some abdominal pain for several hours and vaginal bleeding comparable to a heavy period.

Between seven and twelve weeks of pregnancy, the procedure normally involves a general anaesthetic, and dilatation of the cervix followed by either suction aspiration or curettage, to remove the foetus and placenta.

After twelve weeks of pregnancy, the foetus is too advanced to allow extraction through the narrow vaginal canal. Abortion is induced by various means and the foetus will be expelled, after several hours of uterine contractions, in a recognisable state. This can be a most distressing procedure for a woman (and also for the doctors and nurses attending her).

A small number of terminations are recommended because of the mother's physical health, but the majority are performed for psychosocial reasons, the remainder being performed because of a foetal abnormality detected by a scan or by amniocentesis.

Psychological adjustment to abortion depends largely on the personal circumstances, and the level of support from family or friends. Early abortion (less than eight weeks) generally results in less psychological trauma and regret than later abortions.

Complications of abortion include infection which may spread to the fallopian tubes affecting future fertility, and damage to the cervix resulting in an incompetent cervix and subsequent repeated miscarriages. Perforation of the uterus, although rare, is a major complication.

Therapeutic abortion is a method of terminating pregnancy, whereas contraception aims to prevent pregnancy. Abortion cannot be considered as an alternative to effective contraception.

BETH AND JERRY: Beth rang the NFP teacher for an appointment. She wanted to learn about fertility because she desperately wanted a baby. She found it difficult to talk about what had happened two years ago, without bursting into tears. Both she and Jerry had been so happy when she became pregnant and then the worry of contact with German measles, a blood test, and the advice to have an abortion. Jerry had been a great support. 'It's the only thing we can do,' he tried to comfort her. 'We will have another baby right away.' But now it was nearly two years later and she wasn't pregnant. She dreaded going back to the hospital. Beth started charting, and was reassured by the temperature shift and good mucus symptoms. At the third interview she was more relaxed. She now wanted to talk about the abortion. There were many questions to be answered about the operation, and many fears to be expressed, among others that she might be infertile, and would never have another child. During the next cycle, Beth conceived following intercourse on 'peak' mucus day.

STERILISATION

A couple contemplating sterilisation should understand the implications of the chosen operation. It is the final step, terminating their fertility.

A couple should be adequately counselled, usually by their general practitioner or the doctor who is to perform the operation, to ensure that both partners are confident and happy about their decision.

Male sterilisation by vasectomy

Vasectomy is a minor operation, usually performed under local anaesthetic, which divides each vas deferens as it passes through the scrotum thus preventing sperm from reaching the exterior. Sperm production continues, but they perish at the blind end of the vas deferens. Sexual intercourse is not physically impaired as fluid from the seminal vesicles and the prostate gland is still ejaculated at orgasm.

Additional contraceptive precautions should be taken until two consecutive semen analyses show that there are no remaining sperm in the ejaculate. This may take up to three months or longer.

Vasectomy is an increasingly popular means of limiting a family. The incidence of failure is extremely low, but it may occur if the ends of the vas deferens rejoin. The operation should be considered irreversible.

In practice, reversal of vasectomy may be possible using microsurgical techniques. However, after 5 or 6 years, even if the sperm ducts are successfully rejoined, fertility may not be restored as anti-sperm antibodies are produced which destroy the sperm in the testes.

Female sterilisation or tubal ligation

Female sterilisation is a relatively minor operation, usually performed under general anaesthetic, during which the fallopian tubes are closed, using various procedures, to prevent sperm from reaching the ovum at the outer end of the tube, so that conception is not possible.

Sterilisation via a laparoscope, an instrument used to view the abdominal cavity, has become increasingly popular. It may be performed under local anaesthetic in some centres and frequently involves the use of metal clips to close the tubes.

Pregnancy after female sterilisation is very rare, and can only occur if one of the fallopian tubes re-unites. The operation should be considered irreversible. If reversal techniques are attempted at a later date, for example following remarriage, it is most likely to be successful where there has been minimal tubal damage, for example where clips have been used.

FEMIDOM, THE FEMALE CONDOM

The female condom is a soft, loose, polyurethane tube which lines the vagina. It has an upper ring designed to cover the cervix (rather like a diaphragm) and a lower ring which lies flat against the labia. The material used is stronger than the male condom, so is less likely to break. It is claimed that it is effective against sexually transmitted diseases including HIV and has the advantage over the male condom for some women because it allows them control. The female condom is currently undergoing trials.

Femshield, the femidom or female condom (reproduced from *The Fertility and Contraception Book* by Julia Mosse and Josephine Heaton by permission of Faber & Faber Ltd)

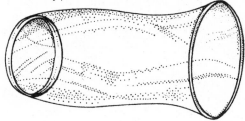

VAGINAL RINGS

Vaginal rings made of soft silicone rubber can be impregnated with either spermicide or hormones. They are designed to remain in place for up to three months. The idea is popular because of their simplicity. Tests are being carried out with various types of this device.

ELECTRICAL DEVICES

Research is proceeding in the USA on an electrical method of contraception. A small long-life battery inserted into the cervix is found to interfere with the motility of sperm and so to prevent conception.

IS THERE AN IDEAL METHOD OF FAMILY PLANNING?

It has been said that the ideal method should be 100 per cent effective, free from side effects and reversible. It should also be cheap, easy to use, unrelated to intercourse, not require medical intervention and be completely acceptable. The ideal method is still a thing of the future.

16 Vaginal Infections, Sexually Transmitted Diseases and Cancer

Information about sexually transmitted diseases is included in this book, because fertility is so easily damaged by these infections. It is important that everyone should understand these health hazards and be prepared to pass on their information to others.

Sexually transmitted disease or venereal disease refers to any infection that is acquired during sexual contact or intercourse. If either a woman or her partner has had sexual contact outside their stable relationship, the risk of acquiring a sexually transmitted disease is always present. Symptoms may be very slight or absent in women, especially in the early stages of infection.

The disease in women may first present as a characteristic vaginal discharge. Observations of cervical mucus will be masked by the infected discharge, resulting in difficulty in interpreting the mucus pattern. If the infection spreads to involve the cervix, causing cervicitis (inflammation of the cervix), then the cervical mucus will also be affected.

A woman who is aware of her normal mucus pattern will be quickly alerted to any change which may indicate infection and she will be in a position to seek prompt medical aid. Treatment in special clinics (found under Venereal Disease in the telephone directory) is completely confidential. If medication is indicated, the course of treatment should be completed as directed, even though symptoms may have been relieved. Abstinence should be observed for the duration of the symptoms and for the time of treatment, as intercourse may cause the infection to spread to neighbouring organs, such as the urinary system, and to the sexual partner.

No one is immune to sexual infection and re-infection can occur as soon as the treatment ends. With early diagnosis and appropriate treatment, most sexually transmitted diseases are completely curable.

CANDIDIASIS OR MONILIAL VAGINAL INFECTION – THRUSH

Most women will experience an attack of thrush (fungal or yeast infection of the vagina) at some stage in their lives. It may be acquired sexually, but also frequently occurs without sexual transmission. Any condition which alters the normally acid environment of the vagina may predispose to thrush, including:

a) pregnancy;
b) diabetes;
c) antibiotics – the normal lacto-bacillae present in the vagina may be destroyed;
d) oral contraceptive pill;
e) poor hygiene – after a bowel movement, the anus should be wiped from front to back to avoid contamination of the vulva;
f) tight jeans, nylon tights and pants – these will increase the warmth and moisture of the genitals;
g) vaginal irritants, for example perfumed soaps, bubble baths and vaginal deodorants – these may cause local inflammation and provide ideal conditions for the growth of yeast.

Symptoms include an intense itching of the vulva or vagina, with or without a thick white cheesy discharge. Small white curds may be seen on the vaginal walls and there may be soreness and pain on passing urine.

Treatment is usually given in the form of antifungal pessaries, for example clotrimazole (Canesten) pessaries placed high in the vagina as directed, plus Canesten cream for the vulval skin. The male partner should also apply the cream to his penis. Some women may have troublesome recurrent episodes of thrush requiring further investigation.

TRICHOMONIASIS (TRICH)

This is a parasitic organism which infects the ridged vaginal lining, causing an intense itching just inside the reddened vagina and a profuse, frothy greenish-yellow offensive discharge. The usual treatment is a course of oral metronidazole (Flagyl) tablets for both partners.

CHLAMYDIA INFECTIONS

Chlamydia are bacteria known to be responsible for a variety of infections including non-specific urethritis and lymphogranuloma venereum – a sexually transmitted disease causing swelling of the lymph glands in the groin. Chlamydia infections are becoming increasingly common. In the female reproductive tract, vaginitis, cervicitis, and salpingitis may result. Treatment involves a course of antibiotics.

NON-SPECIFIC URETHRITIS (NSU)

Non-specific urethritis is a term used to describe inflammation of the urethra of unknown origin, although chlamydia is a frequent cause. The short female urethra is liable to infection from either the bladder or the vagina. It may arise by chance or be sexually transmitted.

Symptoms may include frequent, painful urination, often within twenty-four hours of intercourse, pain during intercourse and possibly a white or yellowish vaginal discharge. If the infection is mild, a woman may be symptom-free. Treatment includes antibiotics for both partners if necessary.

GENITAL HERPES

Genital herpes is caused by herpes simplex virus type 2. (Type 1 usually causes the common coldsore of the mouth or nose.) Genital herpes occurs either as an isolated attack or more commonly as a recurring infection. The first attack, which usually occurs 2–12 days after sexual intercourse with an infected person, is generally the most serious, lasting for 2–3 weeks. Recurrent attacks are usually milder, lasting 5–10 days.

Symptoms include an itching or burning sensation of the genitals, followed two days later by multiple blisters of the vulva, vagina, cervix or rectum. These painful blisters burst in around three days, forming small ulcers with a crust, which heal within 2–3 weeks.

An attack may be brought on by stress, or being 'run down' in some individuals. There may be a general feeling of ill health, with flu-like symptoms, headache, backache, pains down the thighs and a raised temperature accompanying the blisters.

Genital contact and intercourse should be avoided while the tingling sensation and blisters last, to prevent transmission of the virus.

There is no specific cure for genital herpes at present, although treatment with acyclovir (zovirax) will alleviate the symptoms of an attack.

GENITAL WARTS

Genital warts are multiple small growths of skin on the vulva and possibly around the anus, or on the cervix. They are usually, but not always, acquired sexually due to entry of the wart virus through small fissures in the skin or mucus membrane. Symptoms will not be apparent for between two weeks and eight months after the virus was contracted. Effective treatment includes application of podophyllin paint to the warts.

GONORRHOEA

Gonorrhoea is caused by transmission of the gonococcus bacterium during sexual activity. As with most sexually transmitted diseases, because of anatomical differences the male partner is more likely to show symptoms of the disease.

A woman frequently has no symptoms, unless there is an accompanying infection, for example trichomoniasis, in which case the symptoms of this infection will predominate. A woman may have gonorrhoea and unknowingly infect her sexual partner(s). If symptoms are present, they include frequent painful urination and a discharge from the urethra 3–10 days after the infection was contracted.

Treatment usually involves a single injection of a slow release penicillin. If the organism is resistant to penicillin, oral tetracycline may be given.

SYPHILIS

The incidence of syphilis is now very low. It is caused by a spiral-shaped bacterium which leads to the formation of sores or chancres. The sores usually appear at the site of contact. Women are frequently unaware of the hardened, red-rimmed, painless sores, which will disappear within a few weeks even without treatment.

If this stage of the disease is untreated, infection of the blood will follow within a few months. The second stage of the disease, which lasts from 3 to 6 months, will produce symptoms of skin rashes, enlarged lymph glands, fever, sore throat, headaches and many other symptoms associated with generalised infection of the blood and body organs.

If the infection remains untreated at this stage, between 10–20 years later tertiary syphilis will develop, resulting in damage to the heart, brain, spinal cord and eyes, causing blindness.

Treatment of syphilis is with penicillin or tetracycline. If it is treated in the primary or secondary stages, permanent damage will be prevented.

All pregnant women are routinely screened for syphilis (and gonorrhoea) in antenatal clinics, because of the very severe consequences for the developing foetus infected with these diseases.

AIDS (ACQUIRED IMMUNE DEFICIENCY SYNDROME)

History
This was first described in the United States in 1981. At first it was

associated with male homosexuality, but it is now predominantly a heterosexual disorder.

Spread
It is devastating Africa and spreading rapidly in the United States and, so far, to a lesser extent in Europe.

Virus
It is caused by HIV or human immunodeficiency virus. The virus enters the T cells. These are lymphocytes, white blood cells, which carry suitable receptors to attract the virus. These T cells are part of the body's immune defence system to combat infection. Once in the cell, the virus reproduces itself and penetrates the DNA where it becomes a permanent part of the cell nucleus. The virus remains dormant for a variable time, and there is no known way of eradicating it.

Transmission
HIV can only be transmitted by sexual intercourse or by direct injection into the body. Haemophiliacs have been infected by blood transfusions or injections with Factor VIII, a blood product. Drug users can be infected by sharing needles. Very rarely health workers have been infected by accidental needle stab. Mothers infected by HIV can transmit the infection to the baby during pregnancy. The virus can also be transmitted in breast milk. It cannot be caught by kissing, or by using crockery or cutlery that has been used by an infected person. It is not caught from toilet seats and it is not spread by ordinary activities in school or at work.

Course
People infected by HIV react in different ways. Some have a brief illness, similar to influenza or glandular fever, between four weeks and four months from the time of infection. After that many people remain symptom-free for many years and some may never develop AIDS, but the majority become ill between three and ten years from the time that they were infected. Symptoms include profound fatigue, weight loss, fever, night sweats, swollen glands and skin rashes. If untreated the disease progresses towards terminal illness in the form of overwhelming infection resulting in pneumonia, meningitis, encephalitis or septicaemia.

Treatment
People who are HIV positive require support from their relatives, friends

and those around them and they should be encouraged to lead normal lives. There are drugs such as Zidovudine which can slow or even stop the progression of the disease. Appropriate treatment should be given immediately to alleviate any symptoms as they arise and so to prevent debilitation.

Research

There are massive programmes of research in many countries to find a vaccine which will give protection against HIV and also to find new drugs to treat those who have been infected.

HIV testing

Those who have been exposed to the possibility of infection should be offered HIV testing at once and again three months after exposure. The tests should also be offered to their sexual partners. They should be encouraged to have the tests, because in spite of the hardships experienced by those who discover they are infected, there is so much that can be done for them.

Conclusion

In this country there are thousands of men and women who are HIV positive. Most of them are unaware that they have the virus and can transmit it to others. Therein lies the danger. The AIDS epidemic can only be contained if people understand the value of forming stable relationships and act responsibly to protect themselves and others.

HEPATITIS B

Hepatitis B is transmitted in a similar way to HIV. It causes infection of the liver. A vaccine is available against hepatitis B for high-risk groups and gives protection for at least five years.

TO SUMMARISE

Any individual who has unusual symptoms, or who thinks he or she may have contracted a sexually transmitted disease, should see a doctor promptly, or contact the nearest special clinic.

Signs and symptoms related to sexual infection include the following:

a) Discharge from the penis or any other sign of infection in the male partner; b) any unusual vaginal discharge, or irritation of the genitals; c) pain in the lower abdomen – any severe pain, especially if it becomes worse after intercourse, may indicate pelvic infection (pelvic inflammatory disease); d) frequent or painful urination; e) unexplained sores, ulcers, or warts on the genitals or mouth.

It should be emphasised that there may be other explanations for the symptoms apart from sexual infection – for example urinary symptoms may be caused by cystitis, which is very common in women – but medical advice is always necessary for accurate diagnosis and effective treatment.

CANCER OF THE CERVIX

The number of women suffering from cancer of the cervix is increasing. There are certain known risk factors including:

1. Many sexual partners
2. More than five years on the contraceptive pill
3. Sexually transmitted diseases

Certain strains of wart virus, or Human Papilloma Virus, HPV, are thought to cause pre-cancerous changes in cervical cells which are evident on a cervical smear. It takes between 5–10 years from the first appearance of changes in cervical cytology to the development of invasive cancer if the condition is untreated.

If early pre-cancerous cells are detected by cervical smear, a repeat smear will usually be taken, followed by a colposcopy. This is a procedure used to examine the vagina and cervix under magnification through an instrument known as a colposcope. Appropriate treatment will be given according to the findings. This may involve destruction of the affected tissue by cryosurgery (freezing) or laser therapy. If the abnormal cells seem more extensive, a cone biopsy may be performed to remove damaged cells from the cervix and to determine the extent of the invasion. In advanced cases, hysterectomy may be the only effective method of treatment.

ENDOMETRIAL CANCER

There is an increased risk of endometrial cancer (cancer of the uterine lining) in older women, although this is much less common than cervical cancer. Heavy prolonged bleeding with clots in pre-menopausal cycles or bleeding in post-menopausal women should always be investigated.

17 Scientific Research

STUDIES OF CERVICAL MUCUS BY PROFESSOR ODEBLAD_____

Research in the field of infertility in particular has confirmed that if sperm are to penetrate cervical mucus to achieve conception, the mucus must possess certain characteristics.

Professor Odeblad in Sweden has been investigating cervical mucus since the late 1950s. Evidence suggests that there are three different types of mucus produced by specialised parts of the cervix during the menstrual cycle. Mucus production is controlled by hormones, particularly oestrogen and progesterone.

The different types of mucus either impede or encourage sperm motility. The relative amounts of each type of mucus determine the state of fertility (see figure 17.1).

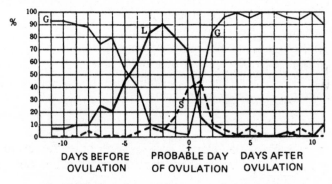

Fig 17.1 Cyclic variation of three types of cervical mucus

Following menstruation, cervical mucus is composed of dense cellular matter (protein fibres), which form an impenetrable barrier to sperm. This characteristically thick, sticky, white/yellow mucus is known as 'G-type' mucus.

As the cycle progresses, under the influence of increasing oestrogens there is a predominance of characteristically lumpy opaque mucus termed L-type mucus. The increased production of the softer L-type mucus coincides with the time a woman experiences the first mucus symptom. That is when there is a sensation of moistness or stickiness and there may be visible mucus at the vulva.

When oestrogen stimulation is at its maximum, a few days before ovulation, the thin, slippery, crystal-clear, stretchy mucus is produced, S-type mucus. The optimum secretion of S-type mucus coincides with the time of maximum lubrication. This may not coincide with peak day which is defined as the *last* day when symptoms of highly fertile type mucus are present.

Fertile mucus is composed of a combination of L-type and S-type mucus. Evidence suggests that a certain proportional balance between these two types of mucus is essential for maximum fertility. Fig 17.2 shows the effect of stretching fertile mucus, known as the Spinnbarkeit test. The uneven thread is due to the presence of thick lumpy L-type mucus along the thread of thin stretchy S-type mucus.

After ovulation the L- and S-type secretions disappear and are replaced by the thick white G-type secretion under the influence of progesterone. This change is observed as the change to dryness or thick sticky mucus following peak day. The post-ovulatory G-type mucus persists until the next menstruation, forming an impenetrable barrier to sperm.

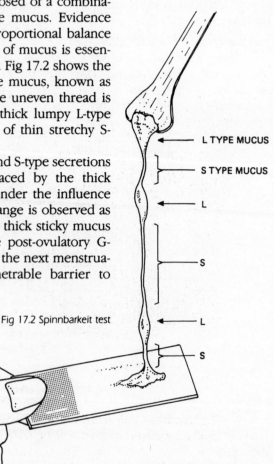

L TYPE MUCUS

S TYPE MUCUS

L

S

L

S

Fig 17.2 Spinnbarkeit test

Observation of the structure of mucus in the cervical canal requires specialised techniques and skills. Inevitably the characteristics of cervical mucus, when it appears at the vulva, will have undergone changes due to the drying effect of the lower vagina and the time taken for the secretions to pass along the ridged vaginal lining.

Samples of mucus taken from the cervical os may be dried on a glass slide and observed under a microscope. Figure 17.3 shows the appearance of the different types of mucus. The L-type mucus is seen as large fern-like crystals hence the name ferning or the fern test. The S-type mucus has thin parallel needles arranged as bundles, and the G-type mucus has irregular shaped crystals or no crystal formation. A well formed fern pattern is an indication of good oestrogen activity and fertility.

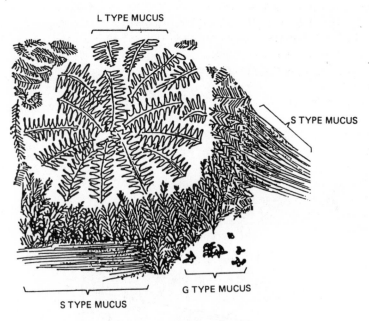

Fig 17.3 Ferning effect

It will be apparent that from the microscopic structure of the three types of mucus, sperm transport will be either encouraged or impeded. Figure 17.4 shows the S-type mucus structure as mucin molecules arranged in parallel bundles with large spaces or swimming lanes between them, containing a watery fluid. This fluid is the natural medium for swimming sperm. In the L-type mucus the mucin bundles lie closer

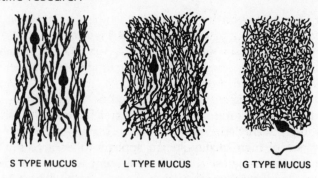

S TYPE MUCUS   L TYPE MUCUS   G TYPE MUCUS

Fig 17.4 Sperm penetration in three types of cervical mucus

together and slow down sperm advance, allowing only partial penetration. The dense molecular network of the G-type mucus acts as an impenetrable barrier to sperm.

The combination of L-type and S-type mucus for maximum fertility has already been mentioned briefly. The alkaline L-type mucus neutralises the acidic vaginal secretions to provide a hospitable medium for sperm survival. It also provides a supportive framework for the S-type swimming lanes. The third function of L-type mucus is to act as a biological filter to weed out defective sperm.

**DIRECTION OF
MUCUS FLOW**

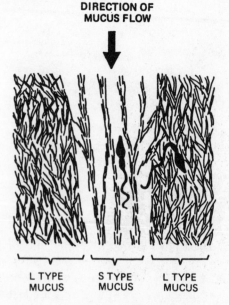

L TYPE   S TYPE   L TYPE
MUCUS   MUCUS   MUCUS

Fig 17.5 L-type mucus capturing defective sperm

Professor Odeblad's theory is illustrated in figure 17.5. Normal healthy high quality sperm swim rapidly upwards inside the swimming lanes of the S-type mucus, but any sperm that are of low quality with abnormal structure (for example broken necks) have an irregular swimming motion. These defective sperm are unable to advance effectively in the swimming lanes but drift sideways where they become captured by the L-type mucus framework (ie the SL mucus system probably favours the advance of high quality sperm).

The advance of high quality sperm appears to be a highly ordered process. It has been suggested that there is some kind of intercommunication system between the sperm cells to assist in the advance of sperm through the genital tract.

Evidence suggests that the three types of mucus are secreted from separate groups of crypts in the cervical canal. Figure 17.6 illustrates the preponderance of S-secreting units in the upper half of the canal, and the distribution of L-secreting units along the whole cervical canal, but dominating the lower half of the canal. The G-secreting units are located around the external os.

The position of the different types of mucus-producing crypts along the length of the cervical canal appears to be a vital part of the whole mucus system. After ovulation has occurred, the formation of the dense G-type

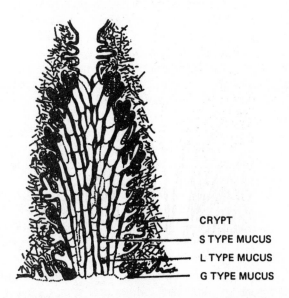

CRYPT
S TYPE MUCUS
L TYPE MUCUS
G TYPE MUCUS

Fig 17.6 Mucus production in the cervical crypts

mucus plug acts to retain any seminal fluid in a special reservoir within the cervical canal to assist in directing sperm upwards towards the S-secreting crypts and the uterine cavity.

The S-type mucus is produced fairly rapidly from crypts in the upper part of the cervix. It flows continuously as long strings of a watery fluid between the L-type mucus framework – this has been likened to water in a brook streaming between pebbles. The continuous flow is necessary to arrange the molecules of S-type mucus into parallel bundles of stringy mucus in swimming lanes.

The work by Professor Odeblad has contributed greatly to our understanding of the mucus system and has generally been accepted and confirmed by other researchers working in the field including the Billings husband and wife team and Professor Hilgers. The evidence to support the validity of the mucus sign as an indicator of fertility is indisputable.

THE CHANCES OF CONCEPTION THROUGHOUT THE MENSTRUAL CYCLE

In the late 1960s a study was conducted by Professor John Marshall and Dr John Barrett to analyse the chance of conception following intercourse on different days of the menstrual cycle. A total of 241 married couples who had proved their fertility by the birth of at least one child participated in the study. The women's ages ranged from 20–49 years.

The couples were using the temperature method following instruction by the CMAC. Other charts were collected by Dr and Mme Charles Rendu of CLER, an organisation based in Paris. Some of the couples were using the knowledge of their fertility to avoid pregnancy, others to conceive and still others changed their intentions during the course of the study from avoiding to planning a further pregnancy.

The women were asked to record their rectal temperature each morning and to record each act of intercourse on their charts. All the data from the charts were computerised. As each couple might have intercourse on several different days in a particular cycle, subsequent conception could not immediately be attributed to a single act of intercourse, therefore a very complex mathematical analysis was involved to produce the results.

It should be noted that in this study, for convenience only, the days were counted before and after the temperature shift, realising that ovulation could not be pinpointed with accuracy.

The results showed that the risks of conception were effectively limited to the five days before the temperature rise and the first day of an elevated temperature. The chance of conception occurring outside these limits approximated to zero.

This study confirmed the impression that the chances of conception following intercourse after the temperature rise are much lower than before the rise. The chance of conception is at its greatest several days prior to the temperature rise, hence the significantly higher user failure rate associated with intercourse in the pre-ovulatory phase.

Using these statistics, a calculation was made to determine the effect of the frequency of intercourse on the chances of conception. If couples are unaware of, or disregard the cyclic phases of fertility and infertility and intercourse takes place at random, the chances of conception will be directly proportional to the frequency of intercourse. Couples who have intercourse once per week have a 14 per cent chance of conceiving in any particular cycle. The chance of conception increases to a maximum of 68 per cent for couples who have intercourse every day.

The results of the Marshall and Barrett study provide valuable supportive evidence when explaining the pregnancy risks to couples or when discussing the chances of pregnancy with subfertile couples.

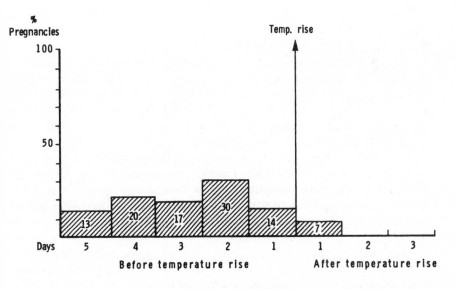

Fig 17.7 Chances of conception

USE OF ULTRASOUND SCANS AND HORMONE ASSAYS TO DETECT THE FERTILE PHASE_____

A study was made in 1984 by Dr Anna Flynn in Birmingham to compare a woman's subjective assessment of the fertile period (by sympto-thermal charting) with urinary hormone levels and detection of ovulation by ultrasound.

The study participants were eight healthy fertile women aged from 25–35 years, who were experienced users of the sympto-thermal method. All the women were asked to observe and record changes in the temperature, mucus and cervix and to note ovulation pain or breast tenderness. Each woman deduced her probable fertile time from these symptothermal indicators.

Measurements of the hormones oestrogen, progesterone, folliclestimulating hormone (FSH) and luteinising hormone (LH) were made using daily specimens of early morning urine.

Ultrasound scans were begun on the day of the cycle the women estimated to be the beginning of their fertile phase, as defined by the first appearance of mucus or S−20 whichever came first. Daily scans were performed to determine the number and size of follicles and to observe ovulation.

When ultrasound waves are directed towards the ovaries, an image of the fluid-filled follicle can be observed. The immature follicle (only a few mm in size) grows to reach full maturity (about 2cm). The ovum is released and the follicle collapses to form the corpus luteum. Ovulation day was considered to be the day following the day that maximum follicular growth was observed.

The study concluded that the most reliable clinical indicator to detect the beginning of the fertile phase was the calendar calculation S−20. Mucus was not always present sufficiently early to warn of approaching fertility, if the couple wished to avoid conception. One pregnancy resulted from intercourse on a dry day (calculated by ultrasound and hormone assays to be five days before ovulation). It was reasonably assumed that if the S−20 rule had been applied, the pregnancy might not have occurred as intercourse would have been discontinued two days previously.

The double check of the first appearance of mucus or S−20 whichever comes first appeared to offer the most reliable combination of indicators. Hormone assays (measurements) did not increase the reliability of detecting the beginning of the fertile phase.

In this study the end of the fertile phase was identified as the morning of the third high temperature or evening of the fourth day after the peak mucus symptom whichever came last. In a minute number of cycles one or other of the indicators (mucus or temperature) fell within the fertile limits defined by hormone assays or ultrasound, but it was considered that using the double check methodology described, very few unplanned pregnancies would be expected.

This study highlighted the accuracy of a woman's subjective assessment of the fertile phase and reconfirmed scientifically the validity of the sympto-thermal guidelines.

Another small study in Cardiff was conducted along similar lines to the Birmingham study. Six women of proven fertility who were NFP users recorded a total of 15 menstrual cycles on sympto-thermal charts. Their subjective assessment of their fertility was compared with measurements of Luteinising Hormone levels and the time of ovulation was estimated on ultrasound scan assuming the day of ovulation as the day before the appearance of the corpus luteum. Three cycles out of the 15 were suggestive of persistent luteinised unruptured follicles.

The researchers commented that the most accurate means of pinpointing ovulation was by identifying the day of the most abundant fertile-type mucus. This was as accurate as luteinising hormone measurements. This finding could be most helpful for couples with fertility problems who wish to maximise their chances of conception.

The day before the temperature shift coincided with the day of ovulation in 8 out of 12 cycles. This was further confirmation of the accuracy of the sympto-thermal guidelines for detecting the onset of the post-ovulatory infertile phase.

The study suggested that when natural family planning methods fail it is not due to the unreliability of the method but to user failure.

DIAGNOSTIC TESTS TO PREDICT THE FERTILE PHASE OF THE CYCLE

There has been a lot of research on the development of simple urinary assays to determine the limits of the fertile phase. The changing oestrogen/progesterone ratio is proving difficult to refine to a simple yet effective home test.

The Progesturine TM PDG identifies the onset of the post-ovulatory infertile phase. It is not yet simplified for use in the home, but could be a substitute for temperature recordings. There is not, as yet, any technological means of determining the onset of the fertile phase in the form of a home kit.

The ovarian monitor

Professor James Brown, who works with Drs John and Lynn Billings in Australia, has developed the ovarian monitor. This measures daily urinary oestrogen and pregnanediol levels in order to identify the periods of fertility and infertility during the menstrual cycle. Testing has been satisfactory and it is hoped that home kits will be made available.

Technological devices based on thermal changes during the cycle

The Rite-time rhythm clock is an electronic thermometer which records and displays the daily temperature and stores the data in the computer. It predicts the fertile phase and the late infertile phase.

The Bioself 110 Fertility Indicator is a similar device which uses a red or green light to indicate the fertile and infertile phases. The reliability of these devices is still not proven.

Evidence suggests that the blood flow to the hands is reduced prior to ovulation, lowering the temperature and closing off the smaller blood vessels. A device which monitors the blood flow is being developed.

Other research projects are currently investigating means of assessing hormone levels in the saliva and in cervical mucus, in an effort to provide a simple, reliable test for domestic use, that will consistently and accurately predict ovulation and the limits of the fertile phase.

Teaching

18 Techniques of Teaching Natural Family Planning

THE NATURAL FAMILY PLANNING TEACHER

Natural family planning is taught by doctors and nurses and by lay people who have attended a teacher training course held by one of the organisations listed at the back of the book. Lay teachers require medical back-up and all teachers require in-service training in order to keep their knowledge up to date. The teacher is generally referred to as 'she' in this chapter because most teachers are women. There are some male teachers working alone and many others who work as part of husband/wife teams.

A teacher needs to be caring and interested in her clients. She must be able to communicate effectively and yet understand the importance of confidentiality. She should respect the unique characteristics of her clients and aim to develop a sensitivity to their feelings. She should not try to impose her own views, moral beliefs or values, but using the skills of a good listener she will identify their needs and so be able to help them. A natural family planning teacher should recognise her limitations. She should be quick to identify those problems which are outside her own expertise and be ready to refer clients to her medical adviser or to other services as appropriate.

Teachers must face the fact that at some time one of their clients will become pregnant – FAILURE. A teacher is responsible for her own standard of teaching, but she is not responsible for the behaviour of her clients. They may depart from the guidelines she has set them for a variety of reasons, such as the difficulty of abstinence, or because of stress in the relationship. Very rarely the method may have failed them.

Whatever the cause of an unplanned pregnancy the teacher should continue to offer support. This can teach a great deal if the couple understand why the pregnancy occurred. It is common experience that many such couples continue to use the method after the birth and find it reliable and suited to their needs.

An unplanned pregnancy does not necessarily mean an unwanted child. Without the support of a teacher, self-taught users of natural family planning are usually devastated by an unplanned pregnancy. Uncertain of where they have gone wrong, they abandon the method labelling it unreliable.

Teaching techniques

Teaching is usually given on a one to one or couple to couple basis, but as more people are looking for instruction in natural methods, programmes for group teaching are available.

All the factual information necessary for teaching the sympto-thermal method of natural family planning is included in this book. Efficiency depends on the experience and skill of the teacher as much as on the motivation of the client. Ideally it should be a co-operative venture between the teacher or teacher couple and both partners.

The first interview may be used to establish background information about the relationship. There may be conflicting views, with regard to achieving or avoiding pregnancy. A couple should be helped to see that fertility awareness signifies the combined fertility of the couple. It is a joint responsibility.

Information has to be tailored to suit the requirements of the individual or couple, and given in accordance with the client's learning capacity. Lack of education is no barrier to learning the method.

Planning is essential. The teaching programme must be arranged so that the subject is covered and each session prepared according to the following criteria – knowledge, skills and attitude.

1. The knowledge is the background information for example the physiology of the temperature rise or the cervical mucus.
2. The skills to be demonstrated include use and care of the thermometer and observation of cervical mucus.
3. The attitudes of the client to the knowledge and skills will determine whether a couple wish more information and decide to use natural family planning, for example a woman may find the prospect of daily temperature taking a daunting one or the observation of cervical mucus unacceptable.

A handout should be given in the form of a book or printed sheet, so that the client always has clear written instructions available.

When interpreting the charts, the colour code – red for period, yellow for fertile and green for infertile can be used to highlight the three phases of the cycle.

During each interview, time should be allowed for questions and for discussion. Clients with family planning, sexual or emotional problems, may find difficulty in expressing their feelings or anxieties and will need time and space to do so.

Teaching resources

Teachers must have access to essential equipment including:

Fertility thermometers
Sympto-thermal charts
Coloured pencils or highlight pens
Record cards
Assessment sheets
Handouts and cards for written instructions
Audio-visual aids may be in the form of flip-charts or overheads prepared by the teacher, or ready-made slide or video programmes.

These teaching aids can be obtained from the natural family planning organisations, the WHO pack or other resource centres listed at the back of the book.

Before being considered autonomous, the client should be asked to demonstrate her ability to:

1. Interpret the temperature chart:
   Length of cycle
   Day of shift
   First day of post-ovulatory infertile phase
2. Interpret the mucus pattern:
   Onset of mucus
   Awareness of different types of mucus by sensation and appearance
   Identify peak day
   Identify the pre- and post-ovulatory infertile phases
3. Apply the formulae:
   Shortest cycle minus 20 to identify the last fertile day
   Earliest shift day minus 7 to identify the first fertile day
4. Explain factors which may affect:
   a. the menstrual cycle
   b. the temperature chart
   c. the mucus pattern
5. Apply the guidelines:
   a. for those wishing to conceive
   b. for those wishing to space or limit the family

LIVING WITH NATURAL FAMILY PLANNING

Couples using natural family planning as a means of spacing or limiting their families are faced with times when they must abstain from intercourse in order to avoid pregnancy.

The word abstinence tends to imply the denial of a pleasant experience. This is a misnomer, as the period of abstinence can be very positive and beneficial to the relationship. Abstinence forms a natural part of every marriage, at times of separation, illness or around the time of childbirth. Nevertheless, abstinence can be difficult, the common problems being sexual frustration and the denial of spontaneity.

Tensions created by abstinence can lead to marital disharmony. It is more likely to do so if the woman alone is responsible for charting and interpreting the charts and if she alone decides when intercourse should or should not take place. It is important that the man should be as knowledgeable about the method as the woman. He should be using natural family planning for valid reasons, such as his concern for his partner's health, from moral convictions, or from dislike of using other methods.

Every teacher of natural family planning should be aware of the problems of abstinence and should therefore make an opportunity for a couple to discuss their difficulties, experienced or anticipated. Those couples who are experiencing difficulties in adapting to periods of abstinence should be helped to find their own way of dealing with the problems. It may be a time for a couple to review their whole sexual relationship. The pattern of sexual behaviour may have to be altered to allow for periods of abstinence from intercourse. Couples should be able to express their feelings about their physical and emotional needs, especially at times when intercourse is not possible. Skin contact, caressing and body massage can be valuable means of expressing love. At times, many women, and, contrary to popular belief many men too, simply wish to be held and cuddled. It is sad that caressing is often almost synonymous with intercourse.

It is worth noting that pyscho-sexual counsellors helping couples with various sexual difficulties, often use a technique first described by Masters and Johnson. This involves periods of abstinence for one or two weeks, with a carefully constructed programme concentrating on loving one another, communicating love by looking, holding, caressing, talking and kissing. When there are no expectations of performance, foreplay in the conventional sense can become a pleasurable end in itself. Following a period of abstinence, many couples report a heightened sense of pleasure in intercourse once more.

Enthusiasm develops among couples using natural family planning. Their communication improves as they learn about their fertility and they grow to understand how they can use this knowledge to plan their families. Every couple has a right to be taught about their fertility and to value this attribute. Using natural family planning, they will be independent and in control of their fertility.

Example of sympto-thermal chart

Name

Number

Shortest known cycle ☐ days
Length of this cycle ☐ days

Route of temperature
Time of taking temperature

O V R

Month
Date

37.5 37.4 37.3 37.2 37.1 37.0 36.9 36.8 36.7 36.6 36.5 36.4 36.3 36.2 36.1 36.0 35.9 35.8 35.7 35.6 35.5

KEY

P	Period or blood loss
D	Dry day
M	Mucus
F	Fertile—type mucus
⊠	Peak day
I	Beginning of probably fertile days
1 2 3	Days after Peak Day

Sexual Intercourse

Days of the Menstrual Cycle 1 2 3 4 5 6 7 8 9 10 11 12 13 14 15 16 17 18 19 20 21 22 23 24 25 26 27 28 29 30 31 32 33 34 35 36 37 38 39 40

Mucus—Sensation
Appearance
Stretch

Cyclical Symptoms

Cervix—Rising
Opening
Softening
Tilt

INSTRUCTIONS FOR USE OF THE SYMPTO-THERMAL CHART

TEMPERATURE

1. Shake the mercury down below 35 degrees C. the night before.

2. Take the temperature immediately on waking, before getting out of bed or doing anything. If the recording time varies by more than one hour, note this on the chart.

3. Either (a) place the bulb of the thermometer under the tongue in contact with the floor of the mouth, close the lips and leave for FIVE minutes, (b) insert the thermometer into the vagina for THREE minutes, (c) smear a trace of vaseline or K.Y. jelly on the bulb and insert into the rectum for THREE minutes. (Any change in temperature-taking route should be made at the beginning of a cycle.)

4. Remove the thermometer, read it and mark on the chart with a dot in the centre of the appropriate square, not on the line. Join the dots to form, a continuous graph.

5. If the mercury stops between two marks, take the lower reading.

6. Clean the thermometer with a little cotton wool and COLD water.

7. The first day of menstruation is Day 1 of the cycle. Start a new chart on that day. If menstruation starts during the day, transfer that morning's temperature to a new chart.

MUCUS

1. Mucus should be observed throughout the day and the chart marked each evening.

2. Mark each day of menstruation or blood loss (including spotting) with a P.

3. Mark each day when there is no mucus with a D.

4. Mark days of sticky white/yellow mucus with an M, and slippery transparent stretchy mucus with an F.

5. Mark peak day (LAST day of highly fertile 'egg-white' mucus) with an X.

6. Use your own words to describe sensation, appearance and finger-test consistency of the mucus.

CERVIX

1. *Cervix during the infertile time:* Mark the cervix as a solid black circle placed low on the baseline, to show a low firm closed cervix ●. Draw a slanted line / below to show the tilt.

2. *Cervix during the fertile time:* Use a clear circle to show the softening of the cervix and an inner ring to show the cervix is open. Place the symbol ◉ higher in the space provided to indicate the rising cervix. Draw a vertical line below to show the fertile cervix straight in position.

SEXUAL INTERCOURSE   Indicate intercourse by placing an I in the space provided.

CYCLICAL SYMPTOMS   Indicate cyclical symptoms for example mid-cycle pain, breast tenderness, abdominal bloating, rectal pressure and mood changes.

DISTURBANCES   Late nights, alcohol, illness, drugs, travel, other physical and emotional upsets, should be noted under the appropriate dates.

For further help or charts, apply to your local CMAC Centre, or to:

The Natural Family Planning Service
Clitherow House, 1 Blythe Mews,
Blythe Road, London W14 0NW   Tel: 01 371 1341

or

188 Park Circus, Glasgow G3 6BE, UK   Tel: 041 332 4914

© CMAC

Addresses

The Natural Family Planning Service
Clitherow House
1 Blythe Mews
Blythe Road
London W14 0NW
Tel: 071 3711341

The National Association of Natural
Family Planning Teachers
N.F.P. Centre
Birmingham Maternity Hospital
Birmingham B15 2TG, UK
Tel: 021 4721377

Billing's Method Reference Centre
Dr Helen Davies
c/o 14 Haslett Avenue
Crawley
W. Sussex, RH10 1HR
Tel: 0444 881744

The Family Planning Information
Service
27/35 Mortimer Street
London W1N 7RJ

Graves Audiovisual Library
Holly House
220 New London Road
Chelmsford
Essex CM2 9BJ, UK

World Health Organization
Geneva, Switzerland

Headquarters of the International
Federation for Family Life Promotion
(IFFLP)
1511 K Street NW
Suite 7000
Washington DC 20005, USA
The Federation is in contact with
affiliated organisations in over 100
countries, and will advise on your local
organisation.

Australian Council of NFP
Department of NFP
Saint Vincent's Hospital
372 Victoria Street
Darlinghurst
New South Wales, Australia

New Zealand Association of NFP
NFP Office
Mater Hospital
Private Bag
Auckland, New Zealand

Serena
151 Holland
Ottowa
Ontario KIY OY2, Canada

Bibliography

NATURAL FAMILY PLANNING BOOKS_____

Billings, Dr Evelyn and Westmore, Ann. *The Billings Method* (Penguin, 1980)

Drake, Katia and Jonathan. *Natural Birth Control* (Thorsons, 1984)

Flynn, Dr Anna and Brooks, Melissa. *A Manual of Natural Family Planning* (George Allen & Unwin, 1984)

Kippley, John. *The Art of Natural Family Planning* (Couple to Couple League, USA, 1982)

Marshall, Professor John. *Natural Family Planning* (Catholic Marriage Advisory Council, 1978)

Menezes, Dr J. A. *Natural Family Planning in Pictures* (Catholic Hospital Association of India, 1982)

Periodic Abstinence for Natural Family Planning (International Planned Parenthood Federation, 1983)

Roetzer, Dr Joseph. *Family Planning the Natural Way* (Fleming H. Revell Company, USA, 1981)

Shivanandan, Mary. *Challenge to Love* (KM Associates, 1979)

Thyma, Paul. *The Double Check Method of Natural Family Planning* (Liturgical Press, 1978)

WHO, Fertility Education Teaching Package (1982)

RESEARCH STUDIES_____

Barbato, M., Bartolotti, M. *Natural Methods for Fertility Control*, prospective study, *International Journal of Fertility and Sterility* 5, Supplement, pp 48–51 (1988)

Flynn, Docker, Morris, Lynch and Roberts, Drs. 'The reliability of women's subjective assessment of the fertile period, relative to urinary gonadotrophins and follicular ultrasonic measurements during the menstrual cycle', *Research in Family Planning* (1983)

Gross, Barbara. *Breastfeeding and the return of fertility*, Endocrine Unit, Department of Medicine, Westmead Centre, N.S.W., Australia. 1983

Keefe, E. F. *Self-observation of the cervix to distinguish days of possible fertility*, Bulletin of the Sloane Hospital for Women, Columbia (1962)

McNeilly, Dr A. *Breastfeeding and Pregnancy* (Edinburgh study of twelve lactating women). Clinical endocrinology. (1982)

Marshall, Professor John. 'A prospective trial of the mucothermic method of natural family planning', *International Review of Natural Family Planning* (Summer 1985)

Marshall, Professor John and Barrett, Dr John. 'The risk of conception on different days of the menstrual cycle', *Population Studies*, vol 23 no 3 (1969)

Odeblad, Professor Erik. 'The biophysical properties of the cervical-vaginal secretions', *International Review of Natural Family Planning* (St Johns, Collegeville, Minnesota) (1983)

Parenteau-Carreau, Dr Suzanne. (SERENA, Canada) *The Return of Fertility in Breastfeeding Women* (Study of fifty-four breastfeeding experiences) (1983)

Perez, A., First Ovulation after Childbirth, American Journal of Obstetrics and Gynaecology 1982

Rice, F.J., Lanctot, C., Garcia-Devesa, *International Journal of Fertility* 26, pp 222–30 (1981)

Wade, M., McCarthy, P. *American Journal of Obs and Gynae* 141, pp 368–76 (1981)

World Health Organisation Studies, *A Prospective Multi-center Trial of the Ovulation Method of Natural Family Planning in Fertility and Sterility* (The American Fertility Society, 1981–3)

1 The Teaching Phase. Vol. 36. No. 2. 1981

2 The Effectiveness Phase. Vol. 36. No. 5. 1981.

3 Characteristics of the Menstrual Cycle and of the fertile phase. Vol. 40. No. 6. 1983.

4 The Outcome of Pregnancy. Vol. 41. No. 4. 1984.

Published by the American Fertility Society, Birmingham, Alabama, U.S.A.

INFERTILITY

Graham, Gosling and France, Drs. 'An evaluation of teaching cervical mucus symptoms to ovulating infertile women', *Australian and New Zealand Journal of Obstetrics and Gynaecology* (1983)

Wood, Professor Carl and Westmore, Ann. *Test-tube Conception* (George Allen & Unwin, 1984)

CONTRACEPTION

Guillebaud, Dr John. *The Pill* (Oxford University Press, 1980)
Loudon, Nancy, *Handbook of family planning.* (Churchill Livingstone, 1985)
Mosse, J. and Heaton, J. *The Fertility and Contraception Book* (Faber and Faber, 1990)
Ortiz, M. E. and Croxatto, H. B. *The mode of action of IUDs, Contraception* Vol 36 no 1, pp 37–53 (1987)

SEXUALLY TRANSMITTED DISEASES

Adler, Professor Michael. 'ABC of sexually transmitted diseases', series of articles in *British Medical Journal* (October 1983 to February 1984)
Adler, Professor Michael *et al.* 'ABC of AIDS', series of articles in *British Medical Journal*, vol 294/295, April–August 1987

GYNAECOLOGY

Bonnar, John, *Recent advances in obstetrics and gynaecology* (1983)
McPherson, Ann (ed). *Women's problems in general practice* (Oxford University Press, 1990)

AUDIO-VISUAL PROGRAMMES

'Natural Family Planning', Parts 1–4, Sympto-thermal method, Breast-feeding, and Pre-menopause programmes.
Tape slide programmes produced in the Dept of Medical Illustration, John Radcliffe Hospital, Oxford, published by Graves Audio-Visual Library, Chelmsford, Essex.
Clubb, Elizabeth and Knight, Jane. *A Guide to Natural Family Planning*, a video in six parts, produced and distributed by the Department of Medical Illustration, John Radcliffe Hospital, Oxford.

Glossary

Abortion The spontaneous or induced termination of pregnancy before the foetus is viable (ie, before the twenty-eighth week of pregnancy).

Abstinence To avoid pregnancy, abstinence from intercourse includes the avoidance of all genital contact during the fertile phase of the cycle.

Adhesion Fibrous tissue that abnormally binds organs or other body parts. It is usually the result of inflammation or abnormal healing of a surgical wound.

Amenorrhoea Prolonged absence of menstruation. Causes include stress, fatigue, psychological disturbance, obesity, weight loss, anorexia nervosa, contraceptive pill, and medical disorders.

Amniocentesis Puncture of the fluid sac surrounding the foetus through the abdominal wall and uterus to obtain a sample of the amniotic fluid for testing. The procedure, performed around the sixteenth week of pregnancy, can be used to diagnose neural tube defects such as spina bifida or genetic defects such as Down's Syndrome (Mongolism).

Androgens Male sex hormones, responsible for the development of male secondary sex characteristics including facial hair and a deep voice. Most androgens, including the principal one, testosterone, are produced in the testes. Small amounts of androgens are also produced in a woman's ovaries and adrenal glands.

Anovulatory (Anovular) cycles A cycle in which ovulation does not occur.

Antibiotic A drug, for example penicillin, that is used to treat diseases caused by bacteria.

Antibody A specific protein substance produced by the body's immune (defence) system in response to intruders, for example bacteria which are rendered harmless.

Arousal fluid The colourless, lubricative fluid secreted around the vaginal opening in response to sexual stimulation, in preparation for intercourse.

Artificial insemination The placement of seminal fluid in the vagina, cervix or uterus by means other than sexual intercourse. The sperm may be from the husband (AIH) or a donor (AID).

Bacteria Microscopic single-celled organisms. Some types of bacteria, known as commensals, live in or on the body without doing any harm and are beneficial to health, eg Doderleins bacillae in the vagina. Pathogenic bacteria cause disease on entering the body, eg gonococcus causes gonorrhoea.

Barrier methods of contraception Any method of contraception which uses a physical barrier to prevent sperm from reaching the ovum, for example the condom or diaphragm in conjunction with spermicidal agents.

Bartholins glands Small glands which produce a colourless lubricative fluid around the vaginal opening in response to sexual stimulation. This fluid is often termed arousal fluid.

Basal body temperature (BBT) The temperature of the body at rest, taken immediately on waking, before any activity.

Basic infertile pattern (BIP) An unchanging pattern of cervical mucus or dryness (and unchanging cervical signs) indicating relative inactivity of the ovaries and low oestrogen levels.

Billings method A technique of natural fertility control in which days of infertility, possible fertility, and maximal fertility are identified by a woman's observations of mucus at the vaginal opening. Developed by Drs John and Evelyn Billings.

Biopsy Removal of tissue from the body for microscopic examination and diagnosis, eg, cone-shaped biopsy of the cervix, for diagnosis and treatment of cervical cancer.

Biphasic chart A temperature chart which shows a pattern of relatively low temperatures in the early part of the cycle, an upward shift of about 0.2°C around the presumed time of ovulation, and a sustained higher level until the next menstruation.

Breastfeeding The process by which the baby is nourished from the mother's breasts. This may take the form of complete mothering, ie total or ecological breastfeeding where the baby is nourished solely from the breasts; or partial breastfeeding where supplementary feeds or solids and a comforter are given.

Calendar calculation, accurate A technique of calculating the early infertile phase based on previous cycle lengths.

Calendar method See Rhythm method.

Cervical crypts Complex pouches in the lining of the cervix which secrete mucus.

Cervical erosion The appearance of the cervix when the mucus cells lining the cervical canal grow over the lip of the cervix.

Cervical mucus The secretion from the cells lining the cervix, which changes under the influence of the sex hormones.

Cervix The lower portion of the uterus that projects into the vagina.

Change of life The menopausal years during which the reproductive function declines and ceases.

Chromosome One of the forty-six microscopic, rod-shaped units that carry the genetic material within each cell.

Chromosomes, sex The chromosomes in the human cell that determine the sex. Females have two 'X' chromosomes and males have one 'X' and one 'Y' chromosome.

Climacteric See Change of life.

Clitoris A small knob of very sensitive erectile tissue, the female counterpart of the male penis, situated where the labia unite at the front.

Coitus See Intercourse.

Coitus interruptus (withdrawal) Sexual intercourse in which the penis is withdrawn to allow ejaculation to take place outside the vagina.

Colostrum The first fluid secreted by the breasts in the last few weeks of pregnancy and the first two to three days after childbirth, until lactation begins.

Colposcopy A procedure used to examine the vagina and cervix under magnification through an instrument known as a colposcope. It is of particular value in the early detection of cancer of the cervix.

Conceive To become pregnant.

Conception Fusion of the sperm and the egg cell.

Condom A sheath of thin rubber worn over the penis to prevent conception.

Contraception The prevention of conception by artificial means.

Contraceptive pill Synthetic hormone(s) taken orally to prevent pregnancy.

Corpus luteum The yellow body formed in the ruptured follicle after ovulation, which produces progesterone. If the ovum (egg cell) is fertilised, the corpus luteum continues to produce hormones to support the early pregnancy. If fertilisation does not occur, the corpus luteum degenerates within 12–16 days.

Coverline A technique used for interpreting a shift on the temperature chart.

Cowper's gland One of a pair of small glands which secretes the lubricative pre-ejaculatory fluid.

Curettage A surgical procedure used to scrape out the surface of the endometrium with an instrument called a curette. The procedure is sometimes known as 'dilatation and curettage' or 'D and C', as the cervix is gradually opened with instruments called dilators, prior to curettage.

Cyst An abnormal sac-like structure containing fluid or semi-solid material, which may present as a lump in various parts of the body. Most cysts are benign (non-malignant) and cause no discomfort, but some may become cancerous, so it is wise to seek medical advice.

Depo-Provera A synthetic progesterone given by injection to provide a three-month contraceptive cover.

Diaphragm A soft rubber device inserted into the vagina prior to intercourse, which covers the cervix and prevents conception.

Dilatation and curettage (D and C) See Curettage.

Doering Rule A calculation to determine the first fertile day of the cycle based on the earliest previous temperature shift.

Douche A cleansing fluid flushed through the vagina as a hygienic measure. The practice is unnecessary and should be strongly discouraged as the normal vaginal environment is altered and the physiological self-cleansing mechanism is destroyed.

Dysmenorrhoea Painful menstruation. Painful spasmodic contractions of the uterus arise just prior to, or for the first few hours of, menstruation, and then gradually subside. Persistent, increasingly severe, or debilitating cramps require medical attention.

Dyspareunia Painful or difficult intercourse.

Ectopic pregnancy The implantation and development of a fertilised ovum outside the uterus, usually in the fallopian tube.

Egg cell See Ovum.

Ejaculation The release of seminal fluid from the penis at male orgasm.

Embryo The initial stages of development of the unborn child from the fertilised egg, to around eight weeks after conception.

Embryo transfer (ET) The transfer of an early embryo that has been undergoing development in the laboratory, to the uterus.

Endometriosis The growth of endometrial tissue in areas other than the uterus, for example the fallopian tubes or the ovaries. A woman may be asymptomatic (sympton-free) or have symptoms of lower abdominal pain, which worsens during menstruation, pain during intercourse and unusually long menstrual periods. Hormone therapy, surgery and pregnancy may improve the condition. Endometriosis may cause infertility.

Endometrium The inner lining of the uterus which is shed during menstruation. If conception occurs, the fertilised egg implants in the endometrium.

Fallopian tube One of a pair of tubes through which the ripened ovum is transported from the ovary towards the uterus. Sperm pass from the uterus towards the outer end of the fallopian tube where fertilisation may take place.

Family planning or birth control The conscious use, by sexually active couples, of methods to achieve, space or avoid pregnancies. Natural family planning methods can be used to achieve or avoid pregnancy, whereas other methods can only be used to prevent pregnancy.

Ferning or the **Fern test** The characteristic ferning pattern shown by fertile mucus when dried on a glass slide.

Fertile phase The days of the menstrual cycle during which sexual intercourse may result in pregnancy.

Fertilisation The fusion of a sperm with an ovum, normally in the outer end of the fallopian tube.

Fertility The ability to produce offspring.

Fertility awareness The sensitivity to the natural changes in a woman's body, during the menstrual cycle.

Fibroïd A fibrous and muscular growth of tissue in the wall of the uterus.

Foetus The unborn child from around eight weeks after conception (when all major organs are formed and it begins to resemble a human being) to the time of birth.

Follicle A small fluid-filled structure in the ovary which contains the ovum. The follicle ruptures the surface of the ovary releasing the ovum at ovulation.

Follicle-stimulating hormone (FSH) The hormone produced by the pituitary gland that stimulates the ovaries to produce mature ova and the hormone oestrogen.

Genetic Relating to hereditary characteristics.

Genital contact Contact between the penis and the vulva without penetration.

Genitalia (Genitals) The organs of reproduction, especially external.

Hormone A chemical substance which is produced in one organ and carried by the blood to another organ where it exerts its effect. For example, follicle-stimulating hormone, which is produced in the pituitary gland and travels via the blood to the ovary where it stimulates the growth and maturation of follicles.

Hot flush A flush is a feeling of heat affecting the face and neck and lasting a few seconds. It may spread over the upper part of the body and be accompanied by sweating.

Human chorionic gonadotrophin (HCG) One of the main hormones unique to pregnancy. It is produced by the developing embryo from its earliest days. Its main action is to maintain the corpus luteum and hence the secretion of oestrogen and progesterone until the placenta has developed sufficiently to take over hormonal production. See Pregnancy test.

Hysterectomy The surgical removal of the uterus.

Idiopathic infertility Infertility of unknown cause.

Implantation The process by which the fertilised egg embeds in the endometrium.

In Vitro **Fertilisation (IVF)** Fertilisation outside the body, in the laboratory (*vitro* = glass).

Infertility Inability to conceive or produce offspring.

Intercourse Sexual activity during which the erect penis is inserted into the vagina where ejaculation takes place.

Inter-menstrual pain See Mittelschmerz.

Inter-menstrual spotting or **light bleeding** Bleeding between two menstrual periods.

Intra-uterine device (IUD – or IUCD for intra-uterine contraceptive device) A device placed in the cavity of the uterus to prevent pregnancy.

Labia The two sets of lips surrounding the vaginal opening, forming part of the female external genitalia.

Lactation The production of milk by the breasts.

Laparoscopy A surgical procedure used to view the abdominal cavity through an instrument known as a laparoscope. It may be used for examination of the ovaries and fallopian tubes in some infertility investigations. It is used in some forms of female sterilisation.

Libido Sexual desire.

Lochia Blood-stained discharges from the uterus for the first few weeks after childbirth.

Luteal phase See Post-ovulatory phase.

Luteinising hormone (LH) A hormone from the pituitary gland that precipitates ovulation and development of the corpus luteum.

Masturbation Stimulation, usually by self manipulation of the genital organs to produce sexual pleasure which may include orgasm.

Menarche The age at which menstruation begins.

Menopause The permanent cessation of menstruation.

Menstrual cycle The cyclical changes in the ovaries, cervix and endometrium under the influence of the sex hormones. The length of the menstrual cycle is calculated from the first day of menstruation to the day before the following menstruation.

Menstrual cycle, phases of There are three specific phases in the menstrual cycle of significance in natural family planning:

1. The pre-ovulatory relatively infertile phase which starts at the onset of menstruation and ends at the onset of the fertile phase.

2. The fertile phase which includes the time of ovulation, and the days before and after ovulation when intercourse may result in pregnancy.

3. The post-ovulatory infertile phase which starts at the completion of the fertile phase and ends at the onset of the next menstruation.

Menstruation, menstrual period, menses The cyclical period of bleeding from the uterus as the endometrium is shed.

Method effectiveness This refers to the effectiveness of a family planning method under ideal conditions, when used according to the instructions. May be referred to as theoretical effectiveness.

Minor indicators of fertility Physical and emotional changes which may provide supplementary evidence of fertility. Minor indicators include Mittelschmerz pain, spotting, breast tenderness and mood changes.

Miscarriage See Abortion.

Mittelschmerz, inter-menstrual or **ovulation pain** One-sided lower abdominal pain occurring around the time of ovulation.

Monophasic chart A temperature chart which does not show the biphasic pattern. The temperature readings will be on one level indicating an absence of ovulation.

Mucothermic or **Double-check method** A method of natural family planning combining the basal body temperature and cervical mucus methods. These terms may be used synonymously with sympto-thermal.

Mucus See Cervical mucus.

Natural family planning Methods for planning or preventing pregnancy by observation of the naturally occurring signs and symptoms of the fertile and infertile phases of the menstrual cycle (WHO definition).

If a couple choose to use barrier methods during the fertile phase, potential risks of confusion and unplanned pregnancy should be appreciated. If a combination of family planning methods are used, this is generally referred to as fertility awareness rather than natural family planning.

Oestrogen A hormone produced mainly in the ovaries, responsible for the development of female secondary sex characteristics, and control of the menstrual cycle. Increasing oestrogen levels in the first part of the menstrual cycle produce significant changes in the cervix and cervical mucus, indicating fertility.

Orgasm The culmination of sexual excitement in the male or female. Ejaculation accompanies male orgasm.

Ovary One of a pair of female sex organs which produce mature ova and the female sex hormones oestrogen and progesterone.

Ovulation The release of a mature ovum from the ovarian follicle.

Ovulation method See Billings method.

Ovulatory cycle A cycle in which ovulation occurs.

Ovum The mature female sex cell, or egg (plural: ova).

Peak day The last day when fertile mucus characteristics are either seen or felt. It coincides closely with ovulation.

Pearl Index A statistical measurement of contraceptive effectiveness, showing the number of pregnancies which would result if 100 women used a given method of family planning for one year.

Pelvic inflammatory disease Infection involving inflammation of the internal female reproductive organs, particularly the fallopian tubes and ovaries.

Penetration The insertion of the penis into the vagina.

Penis The external male organ which is inserted into the vagina during intercourse.

Perineum The area of tissue between the vulva and the anus. The procedure of cutting the perineal tissue to enlarge the vaginal opening and facilitate childbirth is known as episiotomy.

Period See Menstruation.

Periodic abstinence Method(s) of family planning based on voluntary avoidance of intercourse by a couple during the fertile phase of the cycle in order to avoid pregnancy.

Pill See Contraceptive pill.

Pituitary gland The 'master' gland at the base of the brain which produces many important hormones, some of which trigger other glands into making their own hormones. The pituitary functions include hormonal control of the sex glands (ovaries and testes).

Planned pregnancy A pregnancy which is consciously desired and planned by a couple.

Post-coital contraception Emergency contraceptive measure in the form of high-dose pills or insertion of an intra-uterine device, within a specified time following unprotected intercourse.

Post-ovulatory phase The phase from ovulation to the onset of the next menstruation. See Menstrual cycle.

Pre-ejaculatory fluid A small amount of lubricating fluid which is discharged from the penis during sexual excitement, before ejaculation. This may contain sperm.

Pregnancy The condition of nurturing the embryo or foetus within the woman's body, lasting from conception to birth. The normal duration is 265 days from conception to birth, or the more usual calculation of 280 days (40 weeks) from the first day of the last normal period.

Pregnancy test An early-morning urine sample is tested for the presence of human chorionic gonadotrophin (HCG), the pregnancy hormone. A positive result, indicating pregnancy, will not usually be seen for at least one week after the missed period.

Pregnanediol A metabolite (breakdown product) of progesterone, excreted in the urine.

Pre-menopause The period of months or years preceding the menopause during which time there may be emotional and physical changes, including irregularities in the menstrual cycle, as a result of fluctuating hormone levels.

Pre-menstrual syndrome A collection of physical and emotional signs and symptoms which appear during the post-ovulatory phase and disappear at the onset of menstruation. Pre-menstrual symptoms are experienced by most women in varying degrees, but if they become severe it is recognised medically as the pre-menstrual syndrome.

Pre-ovulatory phase The variable-length phase from the onset of menstruation to ovulation. See Menstrual cycle.

Progesterone A hormone produced mainly by the corpus luteum in the ovary following ovulation. It prepares the endometrium for a possible pregnancy. It is also responsible for the rise in basal body temperature, and for the change in mucus to the post-ovulatory infertile state.

Prolactin A pituitary hormone which stimulates the production of breast milk and inhibits the ovarian production of oestrogen.

Prostate gland A gland situated at the base of the male bladder. Its nutritive secretions add volume to make up the seminal fluid.

Puberty The time of life in boys and girls when the reproductive organs become functional and the secondary sexual characteristics appear.

Rhythm method A method of family planning in which the fertile phase of the cycle is calculated according to the lengths of the previous menstrual cycles. Owing to its reliance on regular menstrual cycles and long periods of abstinence, it is neither effective nor generally acceptable as a modern method of natural family planning.

Scrotum Special pouch of skin containing the testes.

Secondary sex characteristics Features of masculinity or femininity that develop at puberty, under hormonal control.

Male – Deep voice, growth of beard, under-arm and pubic hair. Influenced by androgens.

Female – Rounding of breasts, waist and hips, growth of under-arm and pubic hair. Influenced by oestrogens.

Seminal fluid, semen The fluid ejaculated from the penis at orgasm. The viscous fluid contains sperm and secretions from the seminal vesicles and prostate gland.

Seminal vesicle One of a pair of sacs, which opens into the top of the male urethra. Its secretions form part of the seminal fluid.

Sexually transmitted diseases Any infection that is transmitted by sexual contact or intercourse.

Sperm, spermatozoon The mature male sex cell (plural: spermatozoa).

Spermicides Vaginal creams, jellies, pessaries, impregnated films or sponges that can immobilise or destroy sperm.

Spotting Small amounts of red or brownish discharge occurring during the menstrual cycle at times other than the true menstrual period. See Inter-menstrual spotting.

Sterilisation A procedure which renders an individual permanently sterile.

Sterility The inability of a woman to conceive, or of a man to produce sperm.

Stress The reaction, both physical and mental, to the demands made upon an individual.

Subfertility A state of less than normal fertility.

Sympto-thermal method A natural method of family planning combining the basal body temperature and cervical mucus methods used in conjunction with a calendar calculation and the observation of other signs of fertility.

Temperature chart A graph showing variation in daily basal body temperature. See Biphasic and Monophasic chart.

Temperature method A method of natural family planning in which the post-ovulatory infertile phase of the menstrual cycle is identified by a sustained rise in basal body temperature.

Temperature shift The rise in basal body temperature (of around 0.2°C) which divides the early low temperatures from the later, higher level on a biphasic chart.

Testicle (testis) (plural: **testes**) One of a pair of male sex organs which produces sperm and the male sex hormones (androgens) including testosterone.

Testosterone A hormone produced by the testes, responsible for the development of male secondary sex characteristics and functioning of the male reproductive organs.

Ultrasound A diagnostic technique which uses sound waves to produce an image of internal body structures.

Unplanned pregnancy A pregnancy that the couple did not intend and which occurred despite the use of a family planning method to avoid pregnancy.

Urethra The tube which conveys urine from the bladder to the outside. The female urethra is very short, extending from the bladder to the urinary opening at the vulva.

The male urethra is longer, extending along the length of the penis. It also conveys the seminal fluid.

Use effectiveness A measure of the effectiveness of a method of family planning under real-life conditions.

Uterus (womb) The pear-shaped muscular organ in which the fertilised ovum implants and grows for the duration of pregnancy. Muscular contractions of the uterus push the infant out through the birth canal at the time of birth. If implantation does not occur, the uterine lining (endometrium) is shed at menstruation.

Vagina The muscular canal extending from the cervix to the opening at the vulva. Sperm are deposited in the vagina during intercourse. It is also through this canal, that the baby is delivered (birth canal).

Vaginal discharge Any secretion which comes from the vagina, apart from menstrual bleeding (which originates in the uterus).

Normal (physiological) vaginal discharges include mucus from the cervix and clear fluid secreted by the vaginal walls and Bartholin's glands during sexual excitement.

Abnormal (pathological) vaginal discharges are distinguished by their unusual colour and unpleasant odour. They may cause itching, irritation, soreness or burning of the vagina and vulva.

Vas deferens One of a pair of tubes which conveys the seminal fluid from the testis to the urethra.

Vasectomy A male sterilisation procedure in which each vas deferens is cut and the ends separated to prevent the passage of sperm.

Vulva The external female genitalia comprising the clitoris and two sets of labia.

Withdrawal bleed Vaginal bleeding resulting from a fall in the level of reproductive hormones in the blood.

Zygote The fertilised ovum. A single fertilised cell resulting from fusion of the sperm and the egg cell. After further cell division the zygote is known as the embryo.

Index

Scrotum, 14, 15, 186
Secondary sex characteristics
  female, 21, 186
  male, 14, 186
Seminal fluid, semen, 15–16, 186
Seminal vesicles, 15, 186
Sex determination, 24, 71–2
Sexually transmitted diseases, 150–6, 186
Sheath, see Condom
Shift work, 53
Shortest cycle minus 20 rule, 63, 73
Sperm, 15, 16, 186
  antibodies, 120, 148
  penetration in mucus, 27, 28, 125, 159–61
  production, 15
  survival, 17
Spermicides, 143–44, 186
Spotting, 48, 65, 110, 131, 134, 155, 186
Sterilisation, 186
  female, 148
  male, 148
Sterility, 118, 187
Stress, 54–6, 187
Subfertility, 118, 187
Sympto-thermal
  chart, 50, 172–3
  method, 12, 33, 187
Syphilis, 153

Teaching natural family planning, 168–70
Temperature, basal body, 34
Temperature
  factors affecting, 41, 53, 54
  interpreting readings, 35–41
  method, 11, 34–41
  recording and charting, 34–5
  shift, 35–7, 187
Testicles, testes, 14, 15, 187
Testosterone, 14, 187
Thermometer
  computerised, 166
  digital, 35
  fertility, 34
Thrombosis, pill and, 133

Thrush, see Candidiasis
Travel, effect on cycle, 54
Trichomoniasis, 151
Tubal damage, 121
  ligation, see female sterilisation
  surgery, 126
Twins, 24

Ultrasound, 126, 187
Unruptured follicle syndrome, 122
Urethra, 14–16, 20, 187
Use effectiveness, 78, 187
Uterus, 20, 21, 24–6, 187

Vagina, 21, 28–9, 187
  acidity of, 28
  artificial lubricants, 106
  dryness, 29, 106
  infections, 51, 132, 155, 188
  irritants, (feminine hygiene), 51
Vaginitis, 106
Vas deferens, 14, 15, 188
Vasectomy, 148, 188
Venereal disease, see sexually
  transmitted diseases
Visual aids in teaching, 170
Vitamins
  contraceptive pill, 135
  pre-menopause, 107
  pre-menstrual, 68
Vulva, 18–20, 188

Warts – genital, 152
Weaning 90, 93, 94
Weight gain
  menopause and, 107
  pill and, 132, 135
  pe-menstrual, 67
Weight loss, 56, 122
Well Woman clinics, 107, 108
Withdrawal, see coitus interruptus
World Health Organisation, WHO,
  studies, 79, 80

Zygote, 24, 188